THE
LAGUNA
BEACH
DIET

T0145717

THE LAGUNA BEACH DIET

The Healthy Alternative for
Weight Loss, Vitality, and Long Life

BROOKS CARDER, PH.D.

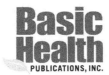

Basic
Health
PUBLICATIONS, INC.

The information contained in this book is based upon the research and personal and professional experiences of the author. It is not intended as a substitute for consulting with your physician or other healthcare provider. Any attempt to diagnose and treat an illness should be done under the direction of a healthcare professional.

The publisher does not advocate the use of any particular healthcare protocol but believes the information in this book should be available to the public. The publisher and author are not responsible for any adverse effects or consequences resulting from the use of the suggestions, preparations, or procedures discussed in this book. Should the reader have any questions concerning the appropriateness of any procedures or preparation mentioned, the author and the publisher strongly suggest consulting a professional healthcare advisor.

Basic Health Publications, Inc.
www.basichealthpub.com

Library of Congress Cataloging-in-Publication Data

Carder, Brooks.
    The Laguna Beach diet : a scientist's guide to painless and sustainable weight loss /
by Brooks Carder.

    p. cm.
    Includes bibliographical references and index.
    ISBN 978-1-68162-812-7 (Pbk.)
    ISBN 978-1-59120-219-6 (Hardcover)

    1. Reducing diets. I. Title.

    RM222.2.C365   2008
    613.2'5—dc22

                                            2007052180

Editor: Cheryl Hirsch
Typesetting/Book design: Gary A. Rosenberg
Cover design: Mike Stromberg

Contents

Acknowledgments

A number of people were invaluable in the writing of this book. Without my wife Fran's success on the Laguna Beach Diet, I would never have even thought of writing such a book. Without her powerful support, I never would have finished it.

My friend Alice Rost, an excellent writer herself, edited and reviewed each chapter as I wrote, providing both expertise and encouragement. Her feedback made this a much stronger book.

It was in a conversation with my friend and colleague Pat Ragan that the idea of this book was born. Pat and I have written several articles and a book together. Pat would have been a co-author on this one, but as a Vice President of a large corporation, he simply did not have time to do it. Nevertheless, he did make a major contribution to Chapter 5. This was like old times for me, as we took many of the tools and principles we used in business, and applied them to the Laguna Beach Diet.

My current editor, Cheryl Hirsch has done an amazing job. Not only has she improved the style, but she has also made significant contributions to the content. When I first saw her comments, I wondered why I was the one writing this book. At the same time, she provided plenty of encouragement.

Finally there are hundreds of scientists, beginning with the late Ancel Keys, who provided the building blocks for this work. I am grateful to them, not only for providing material for my book, but for providing knowledge that is crucial to the health and well-being of all of us.

Prologue

*I*F YOU HAVE BEEN TRYING TO LOSE WEIGHT for years without sustained success, you should read this book. If you want to lose weight but do not want to go through the unpleasantness of calorie deprivation and low-fat diets, you should read this book. If you are happy with your weight and want to stay there, you should also read this book, but it is a bit less urgent. You can finish whatever else you are reading first.

The book has three essential ingredients: First is my personal experience with failure and success at weight loss. Second is my reading of the scientific literature that helped me understand the reasons for my current success and previous failures. This reading convinced me that the experiences that my wife and I have had are in no way unique. Third is my expertise with cooking healthy and delicious food that powerfully supports the process of losing weight and improving our health.

This book describes a method for weight loss that is:

- **Powerful.** I have lost over 12 percent of my body weight and my wife has lost over 15 percent.

- **Sustainable.** My wife and I started this process more than three years ago.

- **Adaptable.** It requires no difficult deprivation, and no peculiar eating regimen.

- **Science-based.** The book discusses the science that indicates that this is the most effective method for sustained weight loss.

- **Healthy.** Not only does your weight go down, but the process also improves cardiovascular health and reduces the likelihood of type 2 diabetes, some forms of cancer, and perhaps even Alzheimer's disease.

- **Fun.** The food is delicious. The book explains how to cook the food and how to find it in restaurants. Success at losing weight is also fun.

It is daunting to write a book on weight loss when there are already hundreds of them out there. On the other hand, most of the methods that these books recommend have no scientific evidence to verify their effectiveness. Testimonials alone mean nothing to me. The more of them I see for a particular product or process, absent of science, the more suspicious I am.

THIS IS NOT A "DIET" BOOK IN THE USUAL SENSE

Let me make clear at the outset that I have problems with the word "diet." Its meaning is frequently misinterpreted. Dictionaries provide at least two meanings: 1) it is the particular selection of foods you eat, or 2) it is a manipulation of your eating regimen, usually involving restriction of calories, fat, or carbohydrates, adopted with the intention of weight loss. The word "diet" derives from the Greek *diaita,* which means "way of life." Eating 1,200 calories per day or a low-carb regimen may be a diet, but it is not an enjoyable way of life in my opinion. The diet I propose is.

This is a "way of life" book. While I cannot guarantee that it will decrease your weight and improve your health, I can assure you that groups that live this way have far less obesity, heart disease, and diabetes than the current population of the United States.

SCIENCE IS THE ULTIMATE ARBITER

The only way to really know if a diet works is to run a controlled study. In a controlled study, a group of people are randomly assigned to either the test diet or to a control diet. Scientists then measure the differences between the groups, using proper statistical tests. Without random assignment, the comparison is not valid. For example, the most motivated dieters might all end up in the test group and the least motivated, in the control group.

While failure of a single study does not prove that the particular diet does not work, it leaves us with no evidence that it does work. If a number of studies fail to show an effect, we can be more convinced that the process is ineffective, although it can always be argued that we just did not apply the program properly. If there are no published studies, we need to ask why. Were the studies done but not published because they were not successful? There is just no way to know. Of the popular commercial weight-loss programs, Weight Watchers, LA Weight Loss, and Jenny Craig, only one, Weight Watchers has been tested in a controlled study. While the results were positive, they were far from impressive. The average weight loss after two years was 3.2 percent of body weight. However, 27 percent of the participants dropped out of the study.

And yet we are bombarded with ads promoting these programs. I am constantly disturbed by claims that are not supported by scientific evidence. I am a scientist and a businessman, not a prophet. I want to make a contribution to setting the record straight. I know that this will be an incremental process. I hope that this book will have enough impact to move us forward a bit.

Sustained weight loss is a difficult proposition at best. No one has found a method that will work for everyone. There are no guarantees. Now I could guarantee that if you eat 1,200 calories each day and exercise moderately, you will lose weight. I would probably be safe to also guarantee that you cannot sustain this regimen. That is the problem with most weight-loss diets. They create loss but the loss cannot be sustained.

The diet I propose may not work for you. You may not lose weight, and if you do, you may not be able to sustain it. But my review of the scientific literature suggests that it is the one with the best probability of success. Even if it were not the best, the food is really good, and that would probably convince me to go with it.

Certainly nearly everyone would agree that most of us need to eat less saturated fat, less refined carbohydrates, more whole grains, and more fresh fruits and vegetables. One aspect of the approach I am recommending, based on the principles of the Mediterranean Diet, makes it very different from most weight-loss diets. The diet includes an abundance of olive oil. Research indicates that this is critical to the success of the program. The

most controversial aspect of the process I propose is that you do not directly attempt to limit calories. The book provides my reasoning about why
this is the proper approach.

BODY WEIGHT IS REGULATED BIOLOGICALLY AT A SET POINT

I majored in psychology at Yale University and continued in graduate
school at the University of Pennsylvania. I focused on physiological psychology, studying the neural control of motivation. Among my teachers
were Professor Philip Teitelbaum and his student, Professor Bartley Hoebel.
They were important pioneers in understanding the neurochemical control
of eating.

Brain science was crude then, with far less technology than we have
now. By making lesions in various parts of the hypothalamus, a primitive
part of the brain, they were able to create obese or underweight rats. From
their research, Professors Teitelbaum and Hoebel hypothesized that body
weight appeared to be controlled by a homeostatic system centered in the
hypothalamus that resisted both weight loss and weight gain.

I call this the "weight thermostat" because the mechanism operates like
a biological thermostat. It is set at a certain weight, referred to as a "set
point." If your weight goes above or below the set point, the mechanism
acts to get you back to the weight at which it is set. Unfortunately, over
time, under the eating and exercise practices of many Americans, the set
point tends to drift up. Exactly why this happens is not clear. However,
diets high in saturated fat appear to raise the set point in both human and
animal studies. Circumstantial evidence from human epidemiological studies shows that a sedentary lifestyle is also an important contributor to raising the set point.

There is wide agreement among researchers that once the set point has
gone up, it is very difficult to bring it back down. That is the most fundamental problem in weight gain and obesity. I never forgot about this phe-
nomenon and learned firsthand about it many years later when I tried to
lose weight myself.

MY BACKGROUND

As an assistant professor of psychology at the University of California at Los Angeles (UCLA) most of my research was in psychopharmacology, using behavioral methods to understand how drugs acted on the brain. I was interested in drug abuse and set up the first graduate program in the Psychology of Drug Abuse, a program funded by the National Institute on Drug Abuse. In an environment of "publish or perish," I did both. While I published a lot, and have continued to publish, I left academia eventually.

Over the years I tired of academia and of trying to raise a family in Los Angeles on a moderate income. After I left academia I first worked for an organization involved in the treatment of drug addiction. Later, I moved into business and managed a marketing communications firm. It was during that period that I met another very influential teacher in my life, W. Edwards Deming, Ph.D.

Dr. Deming was famous as the man who taught the Japanese how to manufacture in the 1950s after World War II. He became a national hero in Japan. The excellence of products from Sony, Toyota, and Honda can trace their origins to his teachings. He was embraced by American industry in the 1980s and programs like Six Sigma at Motorola and General Electric owe much of their content to Dr. Deming's work. (Six Sigma is a set of science-based principles and methods that has enabled dramatic improvements in quality and reductions in cost.) While originally developed for manufacturing, Deming's methods can be used to improve the outcome of any process, including services, and even weight loss.

When I knew him, he was in his nineties and still robust. He delivered a four-day seminar at least every other month; each was attended by 500 to 1,000 people, mostly managers and executives. I attended five of these seminars, one as a student and four as a consultant to teach and answer questions at the breakout sessions.

Deming's genius was the thoughtful and accurate application of scientific method and scientific knowledge to business problems. He thought that four disciplines were critical to management: statistics, psychology, the theory of systems, and the theory of knowledge. My education had encompassed all but the theory of systems. With Dr. Deming's encouragement,

I began to apply my knowledge as a psychologist to business problems.

I have continued to consult and write articles for journals since that time. My first book, *Measurement Matters: How Effective Measurement Drives Business and Safety Performance,* was published by the American Society for Quality in 2004. This present book is another example of my application of scientific principles to real-world problems. Chapter 5 on "Monitoring Your Progress" derives directly from my work on measurement. This chapter provides a scientific approach to distinguish real trends in your weight from random fluctuations.

One of the things that attracted me to Dr. Deming's approach was that he insisted that you needed to get involved with the data. He urged the executives in his seminars to actually plot points on graph paper with pencils. The more general concept was that executives tend to receive reports that are summaries, and the summaries often tell them very little about what is really happening. A classic example of a misleading summary is the old joke about Bill Gates walking into a bar in a middle class neighborhood in which there were already fifty patrons. After his arrival, the bartender notes that the *average net worth* of his patrons is more than 1 billion dollars. This would be a true statement. However, without knowing more about the data, you would have a totally unrealistic notion of the patrons.

To the best of my ability, I have tried to get "close" to the data in attempting to understand diets and weight loss. Part of getting close to and understanding the scientific facts is sharing my own varied experiences with attempting to lose weight. Added to this personal element are the experiences of my wife, who has been very successful at losing weight on this diet. Thus, by giving you the facts from many original studies (not just relying on summaries and reviews), I can use the "hard" scientific data to back up the "soft" evidence of my own successful experience with weight loss. This has convinced me that this process is legitimate, and I hope it will convince you. Finally, I can provide the recipes and information on cooking that will contribute to both the success and the enjoyment of the process.

WHY I AM WRITING A BOOK ON WEIGHT LOSS

About four years ago I began to write a cookbook. I am not a chef, but I love to cook and have no shortage of opinions about food and cooking. I would say I am a competent and creative home chef. My book was going to be called *Cooking Jazz,* because jazz is analogous to my theory of cooking. In jazz, one learns the structure of music (many, though not all of the great jazz artists had extensive formal training). Based on that knowledge, one can improvise and create infinite variety. In cooking, one can learn a set of principles, and then improvise. The principles include some fundamentals of the various cuisines you want to be able to cook. For example, many Italian sauces start with *sofrito,* which is onion and garlic sautéed in olive oil until the onions become translucent. Starting with *sofrito* you can make a pasta sauce out of a nearly infinite variety of main ingredients such as tomatoes, Brussels sprouts, leftover lamb, or whatever else you might have lying around. Most home cooks in my experience do not work from principles and usually stick rigidly to recipes. Cooking this way is less fun and less creative, and the results are not always calibrated to the audience's preference.

I certainly had great enthusiasm about the project, but then the game changed. While my ideas about cooking and my recipes are important to the book, they are no longer the focus. A bit over three years ago, I made an important discovery. Actually, others had made the discovery. I just discovered their discovery. It was a set of principles usually referred to as the Mediterranean Diet. It turns out to be a process for successful and sustained weight loss. That process became the focus of the book. My ability to cook made the process easier and more attractive, although you can engage in the process without cooking if you want.

Though I was very thin in my youth, I began to have a minor problem with weight in my mid-forties. A couple of unsuccessful attempts at dieting convinced me that my weight was indeed regulated very effectively by a biological mechanism that I could not alter. Although I could lose weight for about six months by reducing my calories, eventually I was unable to control my appetite and I would ultimately end up weighing more than when I began the diet.

Since I already knew about the body's regulatory system, the only surprise was that the end result of the diet was actually weight gain. This was not something that was peculiar to me. It turns out that, for many people, the long-term result of diets is weight gain. After my experience with this I made a firm decision never to go on a calorie-restricted diet again. I never tried a low-carb diet, since that made no sense to me. While I did not doubt that it would enable me to lose weight, I did not think I could stay with it, and I thought it would be unhealthy. The scientific data suggests I was right.

The concept of the Mediterranean Diet was immediately attractive to me, since Italian food has always been my favorite. The other thing that was important was that the diet had plenty of fat, mostly in the form of olive oil. When I am hungry, I need something with fat in it to satisfy me. I know I am not unique in this behavior. Both human and animal studies show a shift in preference toward fat as hunger increases.

This is a book about principles of eating and exercise, not a precise list of what you should eat each day. I am suspicious of nutritionists who tell you exactly what to eat. After all, nutritionists used to say we should eat meat every day. Certainly there is considerable research that indicates that our own appetites will often enable us to select a proper diet. Had our ancient ancestors been unable to do this, we would not have survived. On the other hand, primitive man did not face the challenge of ice cream, potato chips, and the Big Gulp. The palatability of foods along with social customs and dietary habits can all influence food choice and interfere with proper selection. If you stick to relatively natural foods, I believe that your appetite proves a very effective guide to what you should eat.

But something has gone awry. My wife and I recently visited the San Diego County Fair, which is within walking distance of our home in the beach community of Del Mar. There are hundreds of food vendors. The leading products are tasty sources of fat and sugar. The prototype is deep-fried Twinkies, which have plenty of both. We found exactly one booth that appeared to have healthy food. I am sure there were more, but they were hidden among the burgers, barbecued pork, cotton candy, ice cream, and curly fries. I did not count how many obese people I saw walking along with a heaping plate of greasy food, but there were scores.

I am increasingly horrified at our national diet, and I live in coastal Southern California, which is relatively more health-oriented than most of the nation. Do not get me wrong, though. This is not a book about tofu and asceticism. I like good food as much as the next person, and, by the way, I hate tofu. But I do want to eat good food that will not injure my health. A simple way to approach this is to find a diet that meets two qualifications: 1) research shows that the people who maintain such a diet are healthy and have low rates of obesity, and 2) the food is attractive to you. The diet that you select under these criteria may not be the best of all possible diets for rapid weight loss, but it can be trusted to work in the long term. The diet I am proposing met those conditions for me. I love the food of Italy. My preference is not the elegant cuisine of Northern Italy but the simpler dishes of Central and Southern Italy. There is a huge body of research demonstrating that the diet of Southern Italy is very healthy.

As I began to lose weight without deprivation or discomfort, my scientific curiosity was challenged, and I began to read the scientific literature to understand what was happening. As I began to see the story unfold, it dawned on me that I should write a book.

I felt that previous discussions of the Mediterranean Diet did not effectively make the case for how powerful it really is. The reader of most books on the topic might be left with the impression that it was simply an attractive and healthy regional cuisine. On the other hand, most of the scientific studies of this diet were directed at the effects of the diet on cardiovascular disease rather than on weight loss. But the data on weight loss is clear. My objective is to tell a story that will convince many more people to try this approach. While it should certainly improve the health of your cardiovascular system, my personal experience and my reading of the scientific literature indicates that this is the most effective route to sustainable weight loss.

HOW TO USE THIS BOOK

You can take two approaches to reading the book. You can trust me and ignore the science. In which case, focus on Chapters 1, 4, 5, 7, and 8. The alternative I recommend is to read the whole book. You do not have to be a scientist to do this, and you will end up with a much more complete understanding of what works, what does not, and why. I believe that this will strongly increase your chance of success in losing weight and improving your health.

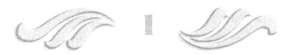

There Is a Better Way: Why the Laguna Beach Diet?

*T*HE SOUTH BEACH DIET was launched in 2003 by Rodale Press. Since then it has sold over 7 million copies. The diet was designed by Florida cardiologist Arthur Agatston, as an alternative to low-fat and low-carbohydrate diets that he had attempted to use with his patients. Because he had little success with these approaches, he developed an alternative. The alternative asserted that there were "good carbohydrates" and "bad carbohydrates," based on the glycemic index. That is a measure of the speed and degree of blood sugar increase following the consumption of the carbohydrate. He emphasized the consumption of natural foods as opposed to processed foods. He also limited saturated fat. While he made some good points, I do not believe that he quite reached the desired destination.

Dr. Agatston argued that his diet was based on science, and to some extent, it was. However, a group of medical scientists actually reviewed his assertions to see if they were supported by scientific evidence. They found forty-two assertions that could be tested. Of these, fourteen (33 percent) were supported, seven (17 percent) were not, eighteen (43 percent) had conflicting evidence with both support and nonsupport, and three had no related evidence in the scientific literature. The assertions that were not supported included claims that: ice cream is less fattening than bread, French fries are better than baked potatoes for losing weight, and fats and proteins cause satiety more efficiently than carbohydrates. Perhaps the most important assertion was the claim that this diet has been "scientifically studied and proven effective." There was not, in fact, a single peer-reviewed study in the literature demonstrating the effectiveness of this diet. That does not mean that the diet is not effective, it just means that there is no scientific evidence that it is effective. Incidentally, as you will see later in the book, few of the popular commercial weight loss programs have been tested in a peer-reviewed study.

The Laguna Beach Diet is based on the principles of the Mediterranean Diet. The effectiveness of this diet is well documented in the scientific literature, having been discussed in hundreds of studies. While it bears some similarity to the South Beach Diet, there are important differences. While both diets emphasize whole grains, and both require avoidance of processed foods, our diet does not make the same set of distinctions about good and bad carbohydrates. The glycemic index does not appear to be the whole story. We accept potatoes and pasta, which are part of a traditional Mediterranean Diet in many areas. We also restrict red meat much more than the South Beach Diet.

We call our diet "The Laguna Beach Diet" for several reasons. While it conforms to the principles of the Mediterranean Diet, as spelled out in detail by researchers, the recipes we offer include Mediterranean dishes, as well as Asian and Mexican dishes, adapted to Mediterranean principles when necessary. For example, I make excellent refried beans with olive oil rather than lard.

According to a 2000 population census, the three largest ethnic groups in this region are Hispanic (40.3 percent), White, non-Hispanic (39.9 percent), and Asian (11.3 percent). Mexican and Asian cuisines are prominent throughout the area. It makes sense then that a Southern California solution would recognize the cuisines of Asia and Mexico. Of course, Italian and Middle Eastern cuisines are also popular in Southern California, and are fundamentally part of the Laguna Beach Diet. Since our diet represents an advance from the South Beach Diet, and because it is very much a diet that originates in Southern California, *The Laguna Beach Diet* is actually a logical title.

As for the scientific validity of our assertions, there is considerable scientific documentation of the effects of the Mediterranean Diet on body weight, cardiovascular health, some forms of cancer, and even on Alzheimer's disease. While many of our dishes are not from the Mediterranean, our food conforms to the scientific definitions of the Mediterranean Diet that are found in the scientific literature. In fact, we provide a scale, developed by scientists, to measure your compliance with the diet.

Of course, the book contains assertions not yet documented in the scientific literature. I have identified these as hypotheses. They are intended to help in understanding how the diet works, rather than to establish that it does work.

THE PARADOX OF OVERWEIGHT AND OBESITY

I know as a scientist that paradoxes can lead to important discoveries. Einstein's theory of relativity is based in part on a paradox. If you throw a ball from a moving vehicle to a person standing still, the speed of the pitch is proportional to the speed of the throw plus the speed of the car. If you shine a beam of light from the vehicle, the speed of the light reaching the person is independent of the speed of the vehicle, no matter how fast the vehicle is going. Unlike the speed of balls, cars, or anything else in our experience, the speed of light is independent of the movement of both the source and the observer. It is always the same from any vantage point. Before you run off to eat a cookie, this is the end of my physics lesson. We are going to focus on a simpler paradox that is closer to home.

For more than twenty years, I have been personally concerned about a paradox in the area of weight control: 1) Our weight is regulated by a powerful biological control system, which I described as a "weight thermostat" in the Prologue. The "weight thermostat" is actually a set of feedback systems in the brain that detect when your weight changes and activate both behavioral and metabolic mechanisms to reverse the change. I will discuss them in detail in Chapter 2. The bottom line is that it is difficult to lose weight and difficult to gain it. 2) About one-third of American adults are obese. While their weight is still regulated by the control mechanisms, it is off the chart. What has happened to the regulatory system? Why is the weight of nearly one-third of American adults regulated at a seriously unhealthy level? It turns out that certain foods, foods that are prominent in the diets of the United States and Western Europe, can gradually move the set point up over time. I will discuss this more later.

The regulatory systems are very powerful. Simply reducing your caloric intake in order to lose weight is usually not an effective strategy. In attempting to do this, you are pitting your willpower against the biological mechanisms that control your appetite. For most people, the willpower cannot defeat the biological controls. It is common for people embarking on a calorie-restricted diet, to lose some weight initially, but eventually gain it all back and more. If you are like me, you have experienced this. I had given up trying to lose weight by eating less. Unfortunately, I thought I had no alternative. Then I found one.

The solution I found is simple and actually enjoyable. I did not invent it. It is based on scientific evidence and confirmed by my personal experience. It will enable you to lose weight without the iron willpower and significant discomfort that are needed to succeed on calorie-restricted diets. This iron discipline is lacking in me, and apparently is lacking in most of us. The process described in this book enlists the regulatory processes of your own body to work for you instead of against you. The result is lower weight and better health. Rather than trying to control your eating with brute force, you can channel it in a direction that is satisfying and healthy at the same time. You do not have to challenge the basic human need for satisfaction in eating.

The reader might ask what my qualifications are for writing about weight loss:

- **Career as a scientist.** I like to say that I am a "recovering academic." I hold a doctorate in physiological psychology from the University of Pennsylvania, and served on the psychology faculty at UCLA. My published research includes papers on brain physiology, pharmacology, and behavior. More recently my scientific work has focused on applications of behavioral science to industrial safety.

- **Experience with inducing change.** Weight loss, under any circumstance, requires behavioral change. For fifteen years I was an executive of an organization that treated drug abusers. For the next twenty years I was a business manager and consultant. I have learned the hard way that attempting to drive change with brute force or incentives is far inferior to using an understanding of the dynamics of the problem. When these dynamics are understood, the solution is often trivially simple. The barriers to weight loss are obviously formidable. An approach that attempts to solve this problem with brute force will fail for most of us.

- **Personal experience with weight loss.** Both my wife and I have firsthand experience with failures of traditional, restriction-diet approaches to weight loss. We have also experienced the benefits of the approach recommended in this book.

A BETTER WAY TO APPROACH WEIGHT LOSS

By the year 2003, I was facing health problems. I needed to lose weight. I knew from experience that a low-calorie diet would not work for me.

My journey to understanding began when I did some casual reading about the Mediterranean Diet, and decided it was time to try it. To set the stage, I will digress a bit. At the time I graduated from college, I was six feet tall and weighed 142 pounds. I thought people who were trying to lose weight were crazy. I wanted to gain weight. Because the regulatory system prevents weight gain as well as weight loss, I could not gain weight, no matter how much I ate. Eventually, years later, I finally got what I wished for and more. By the end of graduate school, I was at a perfect 165 pounds. By the time I reached my forties, I had reached to 180 pounds, and went on my first diet. Though I initially lost weight, like most dieters do at first, I credit that diet for getting me to 190. I can still remember the rebound of binge eating when I went off the diet. I had no control at all.

By the time I reached the age of sixty-two, I began to worry about the 200-pound barrier. I was at 198 pounds. While I was not in the "red zone" of obesity, I did not carry this well. I had had a terrible gut with a 40-inch waist. I was taking Lipitor to keep my cholesterol down, and was having some trouble regulating my blood pressure, even with prescription drugs.

This was not helped by the fact that, by that time, I was an avid cook. Though my favorite food is pasta, I had become very good at pot roast, and also did a good job with lamb and pork. Meat, potatoes, and a salad make an attractive meal that is also easy to prepare. My salvation began with my love for Italian food.

My wife and I made our first trip to Italy in 1999. We traveled through the small towns of Tuscany and had magnificent food. It was usually simple, and with the Euro at about 80 cents, it was inexpensive. The most memorable meal was on the road from Pisa to San Gimignano. Just after passing through a small town, we encountered a line of cars at a rail crossing. Though there was no train, the barrier was down and the lights were flashing. After a few minutes, we decided that this was hopeless for the moment. We had seen a small café in the town we had just passed, and decided to return there for lunch. (We never did ask the restaurant manager if she had jammed the railway barrier.)

When we got there, we found it full of laborers having their midday meal. No one spoke English, but we were welcomed and shown to one of the few open tables. The place was plain but clean, and the staff was very friendly. By pointing to the meals of other patrons and pointing at some menu entries we could translate, we managed to order. I remember the fresh tomatoes, the potatoes, and the simple pasta. It was plain, but absolutely wonderful. With the dollar very strong then, the meal cost less than ten dollars for two, including the requisite glass of wine for each of us.

To us this was the essence of Italian cooking: excellent and fresh ingredients prepared in a very simple way. It was not the finest meal we had on the trip, but, considering the setting and the cost, we remember it best and still talk about it years later. At the time, we did not realize how healthy this approach was.

Some time in 2003 I became aware of studies demonstrating that people who ate a traditional Mediterranean Diet had a much lower risk of cardiovascular disease. Because of my blood pressure, cholesterol level, and waist circumference, I was at increased risk for cardiovascular disease. Therefore, this was important to me. The diet was based on grains, vegetables and fruit, with some fish and chicken, and very little red meat. It included an abundance of olive oil, and moderate consumption of red wine. It sounded like our meals in Tuscany. This looked like my dream diet and, without any more formal study I began to cook and eat this way.

The basics of this diet are depicted in the food pyramid in Figure 1 on page 17, from Oldways Preservation Trust, a nonprofit think tank.

The Oldways pyramid represents actual traditional diets from cultures around the world. These diets have been scientifically proven to promote good health over the long term.

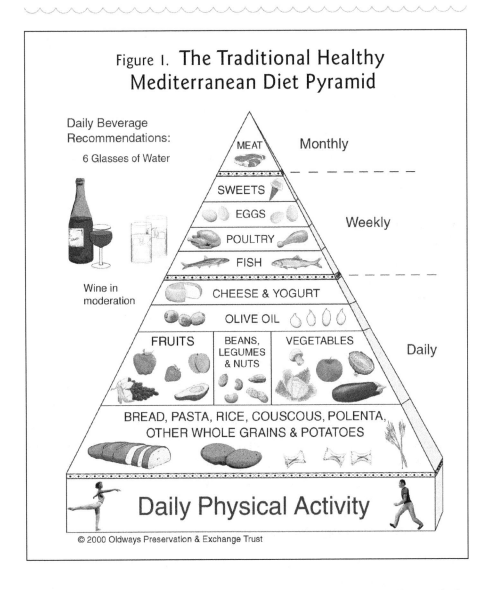

Figure I. **The Traditional Healthy Mediterranean Diet Pyramid**

Daily Beverage Recommendations:

6 Glasses of Water

MEAT — Monthly

SWEETS
EGGS
POULTRY
FISH — Weekly

Wine in moderation

CHEESE & YOGURT
OLIVE OIL

FRUITS | BEANS, LEGUMES & NUTS | VEGETABLES — Daily

BREAD, PASTA, RICE, COUSCOUS, POLENTA, OTHER WHOLE GRAINS & POTATOES

Daily Physical Activity

© 2000 Oldways Preservation & Exchange Trust

To provide more detail on the Oldways recommendations, they include:

1. An abundance of food from plant sources, including fruits, vegetables, potatoes, breads, grains, beans, nuts, and seeds.

2. Emphasis on a variety of minimally processed and, wherever possible, seasonally fresh and locally grown foods (which often maximizes the health-promoting micronutrient and antioxidant content of these foods).

3. Vegetable oils (especially olive oil and canola oil) as the principal fat, replacing other fats and oils (including butter and margarine).

4. Total fat ranging from 25 percent to over 35 percent of energy (calories), including saturated fat, which should be no more than 7 to 8 percent of your total daily calories.

5. Daily consumption of low to moderate amounts (4 to 5 ounces) of cheese and yogurt (recent research suggests low-fat and non-fat versions may be preferable).

6. Weekly consumption (three or more times) of low to moderate amounts (4 to 5 ounces) of fish and poultry (recent research also suggests that fish be somewhat favored over poultry), and from zero to four eggs per week (including those used in cooking and baking).

7. Fresh fruit as the typical daily dessert; sweets with a significant amount of sugar or honey and saturated fat consumed not more than a few times per week.

8. Red meat a few times per month (recent research suggests that if red meat is eaten, its consumption should be limited to a maximum of 12 to 16 ounces, approximately 340 to 450 grams, per month); where the flavor is acceptable, lean versions may be preferable. (I frequently use ground turkey as a substitute for ground beef, and always select lean cuts and small portions when cooking with red meat.)

9. Regular physical activity at a level that promotes a healthy weight, fitness, and well-being.

10. Moderate consumption of wine, normally with meals; about one to two glasses per day for men and one glass per day for women. (From a contemporary public-health perspective, wine should be considered optional and avoided when consumption would put the individual or others at risk.)

There are two things about this approach that disturb many weight-conscious individuals who have experience with attempts at weight loss. First, the diet is relatively high in fat. In fact, the consumption of olive oil is encouraged. Realize that all fats are not equal. Saturated fats, from meat and dairy products, are the problem. Attempting to eliminate all fat from the diet does not appear to be an effective strategy. (Table 1.1 below lists the saturated fat information for some common foods.) The best approach is to replace saturated fats with what are called monounsaturated fats. The best sources of these are olive oil and canola oil.

The other thing that disturbs people is the quantity of carbohydrates in the diet. It is apparent that bread, pasta, and potatoes are at the foundation of the pyramid. Again, not all carbohydrates are equal. Sugars and other refined carbohydrates are a problem. Carbohydrates from fruits, vegetables, and whole grains are beneficial. One of the attempts to identify problem carbohydrates is called the glycemic index. This is a measure of how quickly your blood sugar rises when you consume the food. It is a fundamental concept in the South Beach Diet and the NutriSystem Diet. As I mentioned before, there does not appear to be a single controlled, scientific study demonstrating that either of these approaches works. However, according to them, you should avoid foods with a high glycemic index. Table 1.2 on page 21 lists the glycemic index for some foods:

Fresh fruits and vegetables are usually quite low on the index. Grains

TABLE 1.1 • SATURATED FAT INFORMATION FOR SOME COMMON FOODS

FOOD	SERVING SIZE (ounces)	SATURATED FAT (grams)	CALORIES FROM SATURATED FAT	% OF DAILY SATURATED FAT ALLOWANCE FOR 2,200 CALORIE DIET
Ground turkey	3	2.8	25.2	14%
Chicken breast, boneless, with skin	3	1.8	16.2	9%
Lean ground beef	3	5.6	50.4	29%
Sirloin steak	3	6.4	57.6	33%
Cheddar cheese	3	17.9	161.1	92%
Part skim mozzarella cheese	3	10.8	97.2	55%
Milk 2% fat	8	4.7	42.3	24%

Source: USDA (www.usda.gov)

are in the intermediate range. In whole grain form, they contain fiber and are very healthy. According to the theory, foods over 70 should generally be avoided. But whole-grain bread is nearly 70 and baked potatoes are at 85. But both are fundamental in the Mediterranean Diet. Baked potatoes are especially healthy if you eat the skin. I coat the skin with olive oil before baking, which makes the skin very tasty, at least to me. Something is missing here if table sugar (with a glycemic rating of 65) is superior to whole-grain bread. A much better rule of thumb is to avoid processed carbohydrates and eat real food. Whole grains are good, pop tarts are bad. Whole-wheat bread is good, while table sugar is very bad. If it comes out of the garden it is good, but if it comes out of a factory, avoid it.

Of course, carbohydrates are a source of calories. If you are eating too much saturated fat, carbohydrates will assist you in either gaining weight or preventing weight loss. But if your consumption of saturated fats is low, complex carbohydrates, in the form of fresh fruits and vegetables and whole grains, are the foundation of your diet.

When I share information on this diet with people who have spent a lot of time trying to lose weight, their first reaction is disbelief. The disbelief usually focuses on specifics of the diet. "If I ate all that olive oil I would be as big as a house." Or "I would certainly gain weight if I ate pasta frequently."

What they are ignoring is that the process I am proposing is a *system* of diet and exercise. The output of a system is not the sum of the parts. The parts interact to produce the result. In this case, there is overwhelming evidence that the system I recommend is effective. If people focus on the parts and not the system, they are likely to conclude that it will not work. If you consume a lot of olive oil and/or pasta and do not adhere to the rest of the recommendations, you probably will gain weight. By analogy, when I teach someone to ride a motorcycle, I tell them that they must lean into a turn. The faster they are going, the more they will have to lean. I sometimes get the response, "If I lean over, I will certainly fall down."

That is true if you lean over and are not moving. However, negotiating a turn on a motorcycle is a system that includes the velocity of the bike, the radius of the turn, and the lean angle. So long as these are in balance, the turn will be negotiated successfully. It is the same with the system of eating

TABLE 1.2 • GLYCEMIC INDEX

LOW RATING	VALUE		VALUE
Artichoke	<15	Carrots, cooked	39
Broccoli	<15	Spaghetti	41
Green beans	<15	Grapes	43
Lettuce, all varieties	<15	Orange	43
Tomatoes	15	Canned pinto beans	45
Cherries	22	Long-grain rice	47
Grapefruit	25	Old-fashioned oatmeal	49
Fettuccine	32	Banana	53
Apple	36	Brown rice	55
Whole wheat spaghetti	37		
INTERMEDIATE RATING	**VALUE**		**VALUE**
White rice	56	Table sugar (sucrose)	65
Raisins	64	Whole wheat bread	69
HIGH RATING	**VALUE**		**VALUE**
Bagel	72	Baked potato	85
Corn chips	72	Rice, instant	91
Mashed potatoes	73	French bread	95

and exercise that I am recommending. So long as the system is in balance, it should work for you. If you isolate the parts, it is like leaning the motorcycle when it is not moving forward.

MAIN PRINCIPLES OF THE LAGUNA BEACH DIET

The main principles that have guided me in the Laguna Beach Diet are:

- limit saturated fat;
- avoid processed foods;
- eat plenty of fresh fruits and vegetables and whole grains.

These are a set of principles. In later chapters I will be more specific about how you can apply them in your diet. I am not trying to duplicate the cuisine of Southern Italy, or any other particular place, but I am following the basic principles of the Mediterranean Diet. Many of my recipes have an Italian origin, but others derive from Japan, China, India, and even Mexico. (Mexican food is not usually an easy adaptation, as much as I love it.) Many of my recipes have modifications to fit the principles of the diet, such as the use of olive oil in place of butter, and the use of ground turkey breast to replace ground beef.

Over a six-month period I lost 16 pounds, more than 8 percent of my body weight, reaching 182. I stopped taking cholesterol-lowering drugs, and my total cholesterol remained at 185, a very healthy level. My blood pressure dropped to a healthy range, although I still required some medication. I adhered loosely to the classical description of the Mediterranean Diet, but I adhered tightly to the principles. I ate very little red meat. I used whole-grain bread, brown rice, and other whole grains. I ate more fresh fruit than before (I am convinced that this diet increased my appetite for fruit). I used olive oil in place of butter in cooking. I avoided virtually all processed foods. I ate when I was hungry and continued to eat until I was full. I ate food, often because it was cooked in olive oil, that had plenty of flavor. I drank about two glasses of red wine each day. I always felt satisfied and did not suffer cravings.

My exercise level was and is less than it was in my fifties when my weight was higher. I walk for forty-five minutes about three times each week. I also play golf once each week and usually walk the course rather than ride in a cart. The golf is usually on a hilly course and provides a good workout, though perhaps not an aerobic one.

While this may sound like a testimonial, it is more than that. The successful experience motivated me to consult the scientific literature to understand whether this process would work for others. In addition, it convinced me that this process is not difficult. It is not a radical solution, and certainly not one that required iron discipline from me.

There is a truism in the military that a direct attack is only likely to succeed if you have a superior force. Pitting your willpower against your biological mechanisms for weight and appetite control is an example of attacking directly with a force that is not overwhelmingly superior. Will-power is usually not able to overcome the biology. What ensues is a long and grinding conflict with no obvious exit strategy other than to accept a condition of being overweight or obese that will most likely get worse over time.

The Laguna Beach Diet is an indirect solution. I am not trying to eat less. I *never* think about calories. I eat all I want. I am also not omitting any important food group. I eat plenty of fat, much of it in the form of olive oil and other vegetable fats rather than the saturated fats in meat and dairy products. This indirect approach has worked to reduce my weight and improve my health. More than three years after I started, my weight has continued to decline very gradually, reaching 173 as I write this in early 2008.

My wife has had a similar experience. Since I do the cooking in our home, she necessarily eats a diet very similar to mine. Initially, after I convinced her to try this diet, she wanted more red meat and would order it when we ate in restaurants, which was two to three times per week. Over time her taste for red meat has declined.

When we started, she had a weight problem that was probably partly a result of my previous penchant for cooking pot roast and steak. Because of her weight, she had problems with her back and knees. As a result of our change in diet, she has lost more than 25 pounds, more than 15 percent of her body weight, without the discomfort of food deprivation or a low-fat diet. She still eats an occasional hamburger, but has developed a love of pasta. This has increased the tranquility of our home, since that is my favorite food.

These stories are impressive to me. The most striking things are: 1) The weight loss appears to be sustained. We have been at this for more than three years now, with no relapse or binge eating. 2) The process was painless and in no way did it reduce our enjoyment of food. This is not like snacking on celery and carrots and trying to convince yourself that you love them. Inevitably you will break down and go for ice cream, potato chips, multiple hamburgers, or something like that. With this process, we have not felt restrained and there was no binge eating.

My wife and I recently returned from a seventeen-day trip to the United Kingdom, Spain, and Ireland. We ate well, although none of the meals was remarkable. The diet of southern Spain was relatively easy to adapt to our style of eating. After all, it is on the Mediterranean. However, the diet of Ireland is anything but Mediterranean. Incidentally, overweight and obesity seemed much more prevalent in Ireland than in southern Spain. However, we adapted to the food in Ireland without too much difficulty, eating seafood, vegetables, and pasta dishes and avoiding the meat, gravy, and cream sauces.

During the trip we walked a great deal. Most days we walked over an hour, getting a bit more exercise than we get at home. This was probably crucial to the end result. When we returned home, each of us weighed exactly what we had weighed when we departed.

The message here is that the Laguna Beach Diet is an adaptable process. It is not rigid. You do not have to buy special meals, weigh portions, or anything of the sort. When traveling, you can't really know the recipe that restaurants are using. You need to have the principles of the diet in mind, and make the best choices you can. In my experience, the process is quite robust. You can indulge from time to time without losing ground. In this way it is not like giving up smoking, which I attempted three times and succeeded only on the last try, forty years ago. On two occasions, taking a single cigarette destroyed six months of discipline. This process does not seem to work that way. Many evenings I have a bit of a chocolate bar before bed. My wife orders beef from time to time. This does not appear to cause a problem. I expect that a week of pot roast, pork chops, and ice cream would deal us a serious setback. But I am really not hungry for that stuff these days anyway.

So we appear to have found a process to lose weight that is simple, enjoyable, and robust. It is not arduous or painful. It is not expensive. In fact, the Laguna Beach Diet will likely reduce your food costs. It has enabled my wife and me to lose 50 pounds between us and keep it off. But there is a caution here. While the success that my wife and I have had in this process has convinced us that it works, it should not be enough to convince you. After all, every program for weight loss has at least one success story. The question is, how likely is the process to work for you? That is a question of science and not of testimonials. I will address this in the next two chapters.

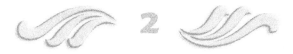

The Weight Thermostat
and the Epidemic of Obesity

*I*F THE ONLY EVIDENCE THAT I HAD was the success that my wife and I have had in losing weight, I would not write a book. I am constantly offended by the ads with testimonials accompanied by before and after photos. No matter what the program is, you can find a few people who succeeded for a short period of time. In fact, psychology tells us that the more difficult a program is to complete, the more enthusiastic a survivor will be about that program. This is why many organizations that want committed members have tough initiation rituals. Someone who completes Marine boot camp is likely to be very proud to be a Marine. Because getting into the organization is so difficult, one then assumes it must be a very good organization. Someone who has survived the discomfort and difficulty of losing weight is likely to be very enthusiastic about the value of the program. What is omitted from the testimonials about diets is a list of the failures. There is a profound *absence* of scientific evidence to support the claims of most of the commercial weight-loss programs, because there are so many failures.

To better understand my own successful experience in losing weight, and to see if this would benefit others, I began to search the scientific literature on obesity, weight loss, and diets. What I discovered absolutely convinced me that the process that I used would work for many people.

To understand the problems of overweight and obesity, and the difficulty of weight loss, it is essential to understand how our weight is regulated.

BODY WEIGHT IS REGULATED BY PRIMITIVE SYSTEMS IN THE BRAIN

Most of us have experienced difficulty in losing weight. Some of us have also experienced similar difficulty in attempting to gain weight. It is as if an unseen force keeps weight right where it is. This is indirect, but vivid evidence that our weight is regulated at a set point, and that set point, for many of us, is different from what we would like. The set point is like a thermostat, except that it controls your weight rather than the temperature of the room.

The accepted science was stated by a recent editorial in a physiology journal: "Body weight regulation . . . is ultimately subject to a homeostatic control system linked with adiposity [amount of body fat]. This control system involves a closed-feedback loop between the central nervous system and the peripheral tissues, whereby the central nervous system interprets a complex set of signals from the periphery and subsequently sends signals to defend a certain level of body weight and fat mass."

To put this into everyday language, there is a mechanism like a thermostat that controls our weight. It has a set point of a certain weight. The set point is defended in two simple ways: If the signals say that body fat is above the set point, the appetite is reduced and metabolism is sped up. If the signals say that adiposity is below the set point, appetite is increased and metabolism is slowed.

Of course, there is not really a thermostat in our brain, but the thermostat is a good model for the biological mechanisms that do exist. Consider a heated room with a thermostat and cold weather outside. If we open a window, the temperature will drop. The thermostat will detect this and activate the heater. Assuming the heater is strong enough, the temperature will return to the previous level. Going on a diet is a bit like opening the window. We lose weight initially, but this activates mechanisms to get the weight back. In weight regulation, the "furnace" is usually strong enough to overcome the opening of a lot of windows. Simply reducing your food consumption is usually an ineffective strategy. To lose weight, you have to find a way to reset the thermostat.

While some of the set-point mechanisms relating to body fat have been studied extensively, it is likely that there are others that have received little attention. In a novel experiment, which could probably not be repeated with humans, researchers implanted small weights into mice: 1 gram, 2 grams, or 3 grams. The implants increased the weight of the mice from 5 to 15 percent. Following the implants, the mice lost weight proportional to the weight of the implant. When the implants were removed, the weight was regained. According to the researchers, "these results suggest the existence of a set point that is sensitive to changes in the perception of mass [weight]. . . ." Thus the set-point mechanism appears to respond both to our fat content and to our actual weight. (I hope this does not lead to the development of weight loss programs that involve the implanting of shot puts into overweight people.)

Let me assure you that animal studies are relevant. The brain systems that control our appetite evolved long before we did. While animal models are not perfect, they are very useful. In addition to implanting weights, we can conduct many other studies with animals that could not be done with humans. For example, we can really control food intake in animals much better than would be practical in an experiment with humans. In a human study, it would be unethical to induce people to eat diets high in saturated fats, given the abundant evidence of the health risks of such diets.

The set point for weight is very resistant to change. Again, according to the editorial cited above: "There is little evidence of an equivalent readjustment of the control system to lower its targeted adiposity level. It is the persistence of the control system and its metabolic adjustments in the face of downward fluctuation in adiposity that explain the most critical problem in obesity treatment: keeping the weight off after weight loss." Translated, it means that the set point is difficult to adjust downward, and thus it is very difficult to lose weight. As you lose weight, the set-point mechanism mobilizes the defenses of appetite and metabolism and the weight is regained. In most cases, losing weight does not move the set point down. This is why it is so difficult to lose weight and nearly impossible to sustain its loss.

Here we have a control system that has evolved over hundreds of thousands of years to defend our body weight. It is reasonable to assume that this control system evolved because it conveyed a survival advantage. It is also reasonable to assume that under most conditions, obesity has a disadvantage in survival. After all, the set-point mechanisms defend against weight gain as well as weight loss. So why is there a worldwide epidemic of obesity?

This epidemic is recent and the magnitude of the problem is very serious. According to the Centers for Disease Control (CDC) in 1960, 45 percent of Americans over the age of twenty were overweight, while by 2002, 65 percent, nearly two-thirds, were overweight. The statistics for obesity are even more alarming. The percentage of obese Americans rose from 13 percent in 1960, to 31 percent in 2002. Nearly one-third of Americans were not just overweight, they were obese.

The definitions used by the CDC are based on what they call body mass index or BMI. The formula is:

$$BMI = \frac{\text{weight in pounds}}{\text{height in inches}^2} \times 703$$

The formula may look a bit strange because the original formula was in the metric system, so the 703 enables the conversion to our English system. To estimate your BMI using pounds and inches, divide your weight in pounds (lbs) by your height in inches squared (height) x (height), and multiply the result by 703.

According to the CDC, *underweight* is a BMI below 18.5; *normal weight* is a BMI between 18.5 and 24.9; *overweight* is between 25.0 and 29.9; and *obese* is a BMI of 30.0 and above. For a man five feet ten inches tall, overweight would be weighing more than 174 pounds and obesity would start at 209. For a woman five feet six inches tall, overweight would start at 155 pounds, and obesity at 186. With my weight at 173 and being six feet tall, my BMI is now a healthy 23.5, down from a high of 26.9.

While the social consequences of being overweight and particularly of being obese can be severe, the health consequences can be even more serious. Again, according to the CDC:

> The BMI ranges are based on the effect body weight has on disease and death. As BMI increases, the risk for some disease increases. Some common conditions related to overweight and obesity include:

- Cardiovascular disease
- Diabetes
- High blood pressure
- Osteoarthritis
- Premature death for obesity and higher ranges of overweight
- Some cancers including colorectal, gallbladder, and pancreatic, along with non-Hodgkin's lymphoma, leukemia, and multiple myelomas

Of course, the CDC adds a caveat:

BMI is only one of many factors used to predict risk for disease. BMI cannot be used to tell a person if he or she has a disease such as diabetes or cancer. It is important to remember that weight is only one factor that is related to disease.

It is also important to realize that being *slightly* overweight is probably not a significant health problem for most people. In fact, people who are slightly overweight tend to live a bit longer. However, when the BMI reaches the level of obesity or even the higher ranges of overweight, the health consequences listed by the CDC are likely to be serious and severe. This book is written for overweight people who want to lose weight, as well as for obese persons, for whom weight loss is a medical necessity. However, people with a BMI in the range of 30, or with serious health problems, should seek medical help in addition to changing the way they eat.

Note that BMI is not the only important measure that relates weight to health. Waist measurement is also important. Abdominal obesity (translated as "beer gut") is a problem. At my top weight of 198, my waist measurement was 40 inches, a very unhealthy level.

Obesity is not just an American problem. Figure 2 on page 30 is from the World Health Organization (WHO), a specialized agency of the United Nations responsible for promoting the highest possible level of health worldwide. It shows the percentage of obese adults in several countries.

This is an area in which the United States is a leader in the negative direction. Over 40 percent of our women are obese. This is a significant increase from the 2002 figure cited earlier. But obesity is also a serious

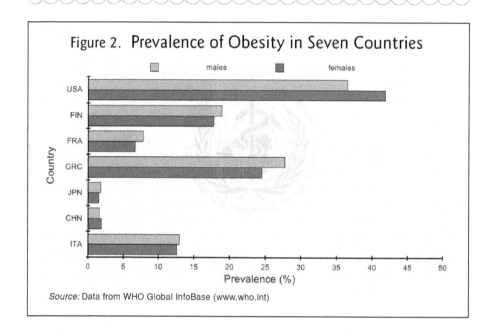

Figure 2. Prevalence of Obesity in Seven Countries

Source: Data from WHO Global InfoBase (www.who.int)

problem in Europe with over 25 percent rates of obesity in Greece. Japan and China have very low rates of obesity. Because of their smaller frame, they should probably have a BMI criterion for obesity lower than 30. Nevertheless, they still have much lower rates of obesity. This is not merely genetic. When Japanese move to America and eat our diet, their obesity rates increase substantially.

The epidemic of obesity continues to increase. Table 2.1 on page 31 compares the data for obesity in males for 2002, to the same data for 2005.

In every case there is an increase. Again, the United States is leading in a negative direction, with by far the largest increase.

Obesity rates in the United States are higher for women, racial/ethnic minorities, the poor, and the less educated. Of course, racial/ethnic minority status, poverty, and lack of education are correlated. This means that any or all could be causes, or even that some other factor, related to these three, could be the cause. What it does suggest, however, is that the development and maintenance of obesity is not a random process. More than that, it can suggest hypotheses about the causes of obesity, although it cannot confirm any particular hypothesis.

TABLE 2.1 • PREVALENCE OF OBESITY (BMI 30) IN MALES BY COUNTRY		
COUNTRY	**2002**	**2005**
USA	32.0	36.5
Greece	26.2	27.7
Canada	23.1	23.7
Finland	18.0	18.9
Italy	12.2	12.9
France	7.2	7.8
Japan	1.5	1.8
China	1.0	1.6

For example, the obesity rate of people with less than a high school education is nearly twice the rate for people who graduated from college. This echoes the rates of smoking, where the smoking rate for those who did not complete high school is three to four times as great as the smoking rates for people with graduate degrees. There are at least two obvious ways that education levels could influence obesity rates. Perhaps more educated people are more likely to see the dangers of obesity and more likely to prevent it or successfully treat it. Alternatively, the lives of the less educated (and the poor and ethnic minorities, and perhaps even women in general) are more stressful. Smoking and excessive eating may be employed to relieve stress. As we shall see later, the effects of stress on eating may contribute to the development of obesity.

Still, the rate of obesity among U.S. adults in 2001 with some college was 20.8 and among "high income" adults was 20.7. Both of these rates are nearly twice the rates for the same groups in 1987. These rates and these trends represent a significant problem. Whatever the causes of obesity, they are not isolated to the poor, the less educated, and racial minorities. And whatever the causes, they seem to have multiplied in their impact over the past twenty years.

WHY IS THERE A WORLDWIDE EPIDEMIC OF OBESITY?

Current theories of why people are overweight or obese include:

- **Many overweight people feel they just have the wrong genes.** We have somehow inherited the tendency to eat too much. Scientists believe that genes do play a role. Over 50 percent of the determination of obesity is estimated to be genetic while the rest is related to environmental factors. This does not mean that if you have the wrong genes, you must be obese. It means that your susceptibility to whatever conditions lead to obesity will be greater. Certainly the genes of Americans did not change dramatically between 1960 and 2002 but the proportions of overweight and obese Americans changed dramatically. While genes plays a role, they cannot account for the epidemic.

- **People just do not care about their weight and appearance.** This hypothesis can be quickly dismissed. It is obvious to anyone who thinks about it that people care a great deal about their weight and appearance. According to the website of the North American Association for the Study of Obesity (www.obesity.org):
  - Approximately 40 percent of women and 25 percent of men attempt to lose weight at any given time.
  - Nationwide, 55 percent of Americans are actively trying to maintain current weight.

OBESITY LOWERS LIFE EXPECTANCY

According to a large prospective study, overweight and obesity have a serious impact on life expectancy. Consider three groups of forty-year-old, non-smoking males. One group has a normal BMI, 18.5–24.9. A second group is overweight with a BMI of 25–29.9. The third group is obese, with a BMI over 30. The first group would be expected to live, on average 83.3 years. The second group would be expected to live to 80.3 years, on average. The obese group would be expected to live, on average, to 77.5 years. The obese group is losing nearly six years of life.

∘ Approximately 45 million Americans diet each year.

But many are taking more drastic steps to improve their appearance and/or reduce their weight. The American Society of Plastic Surgeons reports that in the year 2000, more than 7 million people in the United States underwent some form of cosmetic surgery. Twenty percent of this surgery was performed on nineteen to thirty-five year olds. The top three invasive procedures in this group were nose reshaping, breast augmentation, and liposuction. In fact, we have the paradox of a population getting more and more overweight, yet willing to risk expensive and sometimes dangerous surgery designed to make them look more attractive.

- **Many feel they lack the willpower necessary to maintain a healthy weight.** Many overweight people assume, explicitly or implicitly, that the cause of their being overweight is their weak character or lack of discipline. This is unfortunate, and fundamentally wrong. If bad character is the problem, should we then assume that nearly two thirds of America's population has bad character, or that the national character has gotten dramatically worse since 1960? This just does not make sense.

  The worst thing about this hypothesis is that it leads to solutions based on willpower. The idea is that if an individual is sufficiently motivated, he or she will be able to muster the willpower necessary to reduce their food intake and lose weight. This leads to counseling and group motivational programs, in an attempt to reinforce the willpower of the individual. As we shall see later, these approaches are minimally effective at best, and may even have a negative effect. Many who attempt this approach end up weighing more over time.

- **Eating is an addiction.** This is an extension of the willpower hypothesis. On the surface, it adds no information. It simply restates the idea that a person is eating too much, and that he or she is not capable of curbing this eating in spite of the fact that it is causing serious health and social problems. However, the label of addiction suggests treatment options such as 12-step programs. Our research has found no scientific evidence that such programs are effective for weight loss. However, adding the stigma of "addiction" to the existing social and medical problems associated with obesity is not likely to be helpful.

Other theories have important relevance:

- **We are less physically active than in earlier days.** There is solid evidence that overweight and obese people are less active than people of normal weight. One of the likely reasons that obesity is so much less prevalent in Europe is that Europeans walk much more. Most American communities are laid out so that you have to drive to go anywhere. Most of the European cities we have visited are not this way, although we see more and more congestion on the roads, suggesting that they are probably walking less. If so, this is a bad sign.

  Much of this is speculation. However, there are studies that suggest that moderate exercise can prevent weight gain and more exercise leads to weight loss. However, decreased physical activity is probably not sufficient to explain the dramatic changes we have seen over the past forty years. This may be part of the problem, but is not all of it. Moderate exercise is essential, but not sufficient to achieve and maintain a healthy weight. It must be combined with proper eating.

- **How humans eat has changed.** We have come from a time where we searched for fruits and nuts and were occasionally lucky enough to find carrion, to a time where we have pantries, refrigerators, mealtimes, and nutritionists, not to mention restaurants, take out, and drive-thru. These resources make overeating possible and sometimes probable. We even have social conventions that encourage overeating. For example, for about the past forty-five years I have asserted that parents who insist that children eat everything on their plate are teaching the child to eat when he or she is not hungry. Rather than let the natural regulatory system work, they are forcing the child to overeat. A recent study finally provides me with evidence for this. In a study of 872 children, the authors found that children whose parents used an authoritarian parenting style were *five times as likely to be [seriously] overweight* as children whose parents used an authoritative parenting style. The authors speculated that the authoritative parents allow the children to develop "some of their own self-regulatory abilities." The authoritarian parent might insist that the child eat exactly what the parent thought should be eaten.

  Related to this is the fact that mealtime is often an important social situation. Not only do people feel compelled to attend meals, but often they feel compelled to eat, even if they are not hungry. Again, this is overriding our natural regulatory system.

• **The national diet has changed.** In 1960 I was starting college. My pals and I made the drive between our college in Connecticut and our home in Kansas City several times each year. I recall a McDonald's on the way, somewhere in New Jersey. It was the only one I had ever seen. On the westbound trip, we usually stopped for a bag full of 15-cent burgers to sustain us on the twenty-eight-hour drive. (The Big Mac would not be invented until 1968.) The profound impact of the fast food industry on the American diet over the past forty-five years can be seen from the following statistics:

  ○ Each day, one in four Americans visits a fast-food restaurant.

  ○ In 1972, Americans spent 3 billion dollars a year on fast food. Today we spend more than 110 billion dollars.

  ○ McDonald's feeds more than 46 million people a day—more than the entire population of Spain.

  ○ French fries are the most frequently eaten vegetable in America.

Not surprisingly, there is a study that shows a significant positive relationship, on a statewide basis, between the availability of fast-food restaurants and the rate of obesity. States that had more fast-food restaurants per square mile and more fast-food restaurants per person had higher obesity rates. Before racing to the conclusion that fast food is the problem, you need to consider the following: 1) fast food availability accounted for only 6 percent of the variation in obesity rates, and 2) causation cannot be implied from this data. Rather than fast-food restaurants being a cause of obesity, it may be that a high rate of obesity leads to the opening of more fast-food restaurants in an area. Alternatively, both obesity rates and the density of fast-food restaurants are both related to some other variable, like a cultural preference for foods that are high in fat.

While fast food may not be the sole culprit, it is certainly part of the problem. Much, but not all, fast food is very high in saturated fats and refined carbohydrates. A 42-ounce super-sized soda contains more than 500 calories and more than 25 teaspoons of sugar. If you consume fast-food hamburgers and sodas frequently, you are likely to have a weight problem. However, simply eliminating fast food from your diet will probably not lead to substantial weight loss.

Fast food is only one dimension of the change in our diet. We eat more meat, more processed foods, more refined carbohydrates, and less fresh fruit and vegetables.

Perhaps even more important than the advent of fast food has been the introduction of very large quantities of high-fructose corn syrup (HFCS) into the American diet. This is now the principle sweetener in processed foods and sweetened beverages, replacing sucrose from cane sugar, which is more expensive. While the caloric content of both sweeteners is high, their impact on metabolism is different. Apparently, the liver has a problem handling large quantities of fructose, which leads to increased triglycerides and cholesterol, along with insulin resistance, a precursor to type 2 diabetes. A group of biochemists has recently concluded that "the alarming increase in fructose consumption [via HFCS] may be an important contributor to the epidemic of diabetes and insulin resistant diabetes in both pediatric and adult populations."

You will see that all of these changes are important. I believe that these changes in our diet are the largest part of the problem.

The President's Cancer Panel recently issued its report for 2006/2007. The panel highlighted the relationship between diet and obesity and diseases related to obesity, including diabetes, high blood pressure, heart disease, high cholesterol, and of course, cancer. They faulted government agricultural policy as an important contributor: "We [the U.S. government] heavily subsidize the growth of foods (e.g., corn, soy) that in their processed forms (e.g., high-fructose corn syrup, hydrogenated corn and soybean oils, grain-fed cattle) are known contributors to obesity and associated chronic diseases, including cancer." The panel goes on to recommend that Congress: "Structure farm supports to incentivize/encourage increased production of fruits and vegetables; limit farm subsidies that promote the production of high-fructose corn syrup for use in food."

This certainly reinforces the assertions made in this chapter. (Incidentally, they also cite lack of exercise as a causative factor of cancer.) The report provides powerful support for public health advocates in a struggle against the vast resources of the food industry and farm lobby. As of this writing, the report has not received wide publicity, but I expect it will receive increasing attention.

IS HIGH-FRUCTOSE CORN SYRUP (HFCS) REALLY A PROBLEM?

In an interesting article, George Bray, the founder of the North American Association for the Study of Obesity, points out that the increase in American consumption of HFCS from 1970 to 2000, particularly in sweetened beverages, parallels a dramatic increase in the prevalence of obesity over the same period. Based on the metabolic effects of fructose, he argues that there is a causal relationship. Fructose does not create the usual signals of satiety, and fructose is metabolized into lipids. Thus he sees HFCS as a major culprit.

In an excellent critique of the paper, Michael Jacobson of the Center for Science in the Public Interest argues that the observation of a rise in obesity happening at the same time as a rise in consumption of HFCS does not imply causation. He also notes that the body ultimately obtains as much fructose from sucrose (table sugar), the sweetener that HFCS replaced, as it does from HFCS. He is not arguing that there is no problem with fructose, but that if we replaced all the HFCS with sucrose, we would still have the same problem.

He cites the following as more likely causative factors in the obesity epidemic: 1) massive advertising and promotion by the soft drink industry which have led to dramatic increases in consumption; 2) serving sizes that have increased from 6.5 ounces to as much as 64 ounces; 3) soft drinks becoming a standard beverage for children at fast-food restaurants; 4) huge servings at movies and convenience stores; and 5) wide presence of soft-drink vending machines.

HOW DIET INFLUENCES THE SET POINT

I have briefly described the set-point mechanism, and offered the hypothesis that our set points have been raised by the dietary changes in the United States and Western Europe. A review of the scientific literature indicates the following:

1. Populations that eat diets that are low in saturated fat (such as the fat from meat and dairy products) have a lower set point, that is, less obesity.

2. When these populations change their diet to include more saturated fat, obesity increases, indicating that the set point has gone up.

3. In animal studies the introduction of a diet high in saturated fats increases the set point.

The availability of saturated fat appears to be crucial. In poor societies, where saturated fat is an expensive luxury, obesity is rare, and usually found only among the rich. In affluent societies, where everyone can afford plenty of saturated fat, obesity is common but the poor are fatter than the rich.

The classic study of populations and diet is the "Seven Countries Study" conducted by Ancel Keys, Ph.D., and his colleagues in the late 1950s and early 1960s. While the original study focused on deaths from heart disease, later work confirms that BMI correlates with death from cardiovascular disease. As BMI goes up, so do cardiovascular deaths. Keys and his colleagues studied more than 12,000 men in sixteen groups in seven countries. They evaluated what these groups ate, and measured deaths from coronary heart disease over a twenty-five-year period. The lowest death rates were in Japan, Southern Italy, and Crete. The highest rates were in Finland, five times as high. Finland was closely followed by the United States, with a rate about four times as high as the Japanese and Mediterranean groups. Subsequent analysis demonstrated that the strongest predictor of death from coronary heart disease was the consumption of saturated fat, such as the fat found in red meat and dairy products.

The epidemiological evidence points to the conclusion that our set point increases in the presence of increased saturated fat.

Controlled animal studies have also shown that a high-fat diet can raise the set point for body mass. In fact, these animal studies demonstrate that the kind of fat in a high-fat diet does make a difference. High-fat diets consisting of beef fat cause much more weight gain that high-fat diets made with canola oil or fish oil, although the caloric density is essentially the same.

A powerful bit of evidence that high-fat consumption plays a role in the development of obesity comes from a study of pairs of identical twins where one member of the pair was normal and one was obese. A single environmental factor appears to have been responsible. Every pair reported that the obese twin showed a preference for fatty foods early in life. Since the genetics of the two members of each pair are identical, the cause of the obesity of one twin must be environmental. It appears that this environmental cause is the excess consumption of saturated fat. Of course, this leaves the question of why one twin had a stronger preference for saturated fat. Since the genetics were the same, this attraction to fatty foods must have come from some environmental factor that was not identified in the study.

The bottom line appears to be that our decrease in exercise and our increased consumption of saturated fats has led to a dramatic upward shift in the weight thermostats of millions of people. The availability of sugar and refined carbohydrates has helped to fuel the resulting weight gain. For most, this shift is not temporary. While many can lose weight in the short term, the long-term prognosis has been very poor. In the next chapter I will discuss some of the problems that are inherent in the most common approaches to weight loss.

Combating the Obesity Epidemic:
What Works and What Doesn't

W EIGHT LOSS IS A BIG BUSINESS in the United States. According to the website of the North American Association for the Study of Obesity (www.obesity.org):

- Consumers spend about 30 billion dollars per year trying to lose weight or prevent weight gain. This figure includes spending on diet sodas, diet foods, artificially sweetened products, appetite suppressants, diet books, videos and cassettes, medically supervised and commercial programs, and fitness clubs.

- Spending on weight loss programs is estimated at 1 to 2 billion dollars per year.

It is obvious from the continuing development of the obesity epidemic, that this expenditure is not having the desired impact.

Scientific study reinforces this conclusion. In a review of major commercial weight-loss programs that appeared in the *Annals of Internal Medicine* in 2005, the authors reported that only one mass-market program, Weight Watchers, has been studied in a controlled trial. The maximum average weight loss was 5.3 percent of body weight at six months, with an average loss of 3.2 percent at a two-year follow-up. This is for the people who stayed with the program. The attrition rate was 27 percent. The study found that "commercial interventions available over the Internet and organized self-help programs produced minimal weight loss." More weight loss, as much as 15 to 25 percent of body weight, for obese individuals was produced by medically supervised programs, but the authors point out that "these programs were associated with high costs, high attrition rates, and a high probability of regaining 50 percent or more of the lost weight in one to two years."

The diets tested all involve reduced caloric intake, and many also have a reduction in the proportion of calories from fat. There are problems with both of these approaches as I discuss below.

THE OBVIOUS SOLUTIONS HAVE UNINTENDED EFFECTS

If high-fat diets lead to overweight and obesity, it should follow that low-fat diets would be an appropriate approach to weight loss. In fact, the National Institutes of Health's (NIH) position paper on treatment of overweight and obesity recommends fat reduction, although not extreme reduction. It suggests that less than 30 percent of the energy (calories) come from dietary fat. In the executive summary, it says nothing about what kind of fat. The NIH paper also points out that a reduction in caloric intake is necessary, and that moderate exercise is important. This sounds simple.

Most authorities would agree that you will have to eat fewer calories to lose weight. An exception comes from *The China Study* (Benbella Books, 2004), in which the authors describe a Chinese group eating 30 percent more calories than a comparison group of Americans but weighing 20 percent less. The authors' explanation is that the Americans, eating a high-fat, high-protein diet, are retaining more calories than the Chinese.

WHAT IS A CALORIE?

A calorie, in the context of nutrition, is a measure of energy. One calorie is the amount of energy required to raise the temperature of one kilogram (one liter) of water by 1°C. The caloric content of a portion of food then, represents the amount of energy released when the food is utilized in the body. One gram of carbohydrate or protein contains four calories, while one gram of fat contains nine calories.

Even if you do have to ultimately reduce your caloric intake, the direct approach has problems. Programs that limit caloric intake and fat consumption do not have much success in creating sustained weight loss. Weight Watchers, the only large program that has been tested in a controlled trial, is a low-calorie, low-fat diet. Remember that the average weight loss for those that stayed in the study, after two years, was 3.2 percent of body weight. The people in these studies had BMIs averaging over 33. Thus, after two years of Weight Watchers they still had an average BMI over 30, meaning that they would still be obese.

To put this in real numbers, a woman (or man) five feet six inches tall and weighing 204 pounds would have a BMI of about 33. After losing 3.2 percent of body weight, or about 6.5 pounds, she would have a BMI of 31.9. And this is for the participants who remained in the program. Of course, this is the average. In the largest Weight Watchers's study, the most successful participant had a weight loss of 62 pounds while the least successful *gained* 26 pounds. Sixteen percent of the participants lost over 10 percent of their body weight and 62 percent lost some weight, while 38 percent gained weight, in spite of remaining in the program. While the program worked for some it does not look like a promising approach for most of us. This should not be taken as an indictment of Weight Watchers. Their program was more effective than the comparison group, and they should be strongly commended for submitting their program to a controlled trial, published in a peer-reviewed journal. To my knowledge, this has not been done by the other large programs, Jenny Craig and LA Weight Loss.

If one could remain on a reduced-calorie, low-fat diet indefinitely, one could maintain significant weight loss. However, these diets are activating the set-point mechanisms that slow metabolism and powerfully increase appetite. In addition, there are at least two more problems with low-fat diets: 1) they reduce HDL (good) cholesterol, and 2) more important, they are not very palatable. My unpleasant experience on low-fat diets is one of increasing desperation to taste the deeper flavor that is associated with fats. The longer you stay with the diet, the less satisfying the meals. This is a powerful reason why people have difficulty staying on low-fat diets.

This lack of palatability probably explains the result of a recent controlled experiment. The subjects were French patients who were attending a center for detection and prevention of arteriosclerosis. One group was placed on a low-fat diet, with less than 30 percent of calories from fat. The other was placed on a Mediterranean Diet with fat accounting for 35 to 38 percent of calories, and the further stipulation that 50 percent of fat calories were to be from monounsaturated fat (such as olive oil). The Mediterranean-diet group was allowed red wine, while the low-fat group was asked to avoid alcohol.

After three months, both groups had lost a moderate amount of weight, with no difference between the groups for those remaining in the study. Both groups had reduced their cardiovascular risk factors, with the Mediterranean-diet group having a greater reduction. But most important, 36 percent of the low-fat group dropped out over the three months, while only 16 percent of the Mediterranean-diet group dropped out, a difference that is statistically significant. Obviously, the Mediterranean Diet was superior in this trial, not because it was more effective in reducing weight, but rather because it was more sustainable. Because the low-fat diet was not extreme, there was no effect on HDL cholesterol, though this effect has been observed in many studies with lower fat levels.

Additional important evidence on the limitations of low-fat diets comes from a study of formerly obese individuals who had maintained significant weight loss for over three years. They were compared to obese individuals who had lost significant weight and regained it as well as to a group of obese people who had never lost significant weight. Analysis showed that the weight loss maintainers were not more likely to employ calorie-controlled diets or low-fat diets than the regainers or the stable obese. The authors noted that while calorie-controlled diets promote initial weight loss, they also appear to promote subsequent weight gain. The one dietary habit that differentiated the maintainers was that they were more likely than the other two groups to employ what the researchers called "healthy eating." While the authors did not define this, this has been defined elsewhere as a diet high in whole grains, fresh fruits, and vegetables, and low in saturated fat, but not low in overall fat, a diet very similar to the Mediterranean Diet.

Thus, while reduction of fat in the diet would seem to be a logical approach to weight loss, it does not appear to be a very effective strategy. Of course, a reduction in total calories eaten will also lead to weight loss. But there appear to be limitations to this strategy as well, as suggested by the study mentioned above. Formerly obese people who were able to maintain their weight loss were not more likely to use reduced calorie diets than groups who could not lose weight or lost weight and then regained it.

The strongest limitation of reduced calorie diets is that they are un-pleasant, in proportion to the degree to which intake is reduced below the level of appetite. It is not surprising that the body would be prepared to defend itself against food deprivation. It does so by reducing metabolic rate to conserve energy and by increasing appetite and the motivation to obtain food. The only surprising thing about the process is that in overweight and obese people, these mechanisms are effectively defending a set point that is unhealthy.

It should be obvious that our appetites are largely outside the control of our conscious minds. If this were not so, weight loss would not be difficult. For example, the thought that a low-calorie diet would be good for us does not have an impact on our appetite. We may adopt it for a time, but we do not like it.

Many of us have experienced a vivid example of the lack of conscious control of appetite by developing food aversions. If you eat a somewhat novel food (something you eat occasionally at most) and then get sick, you will develop an aversion to that food even if you are absolutely certain that the food had nothing to do with your illness. Once when I was in college, I ate a Chinese meal and then took some medicine that evening. I know it was the medicine that made me sick, but even the smell of Chinese food made me nauseous for the next ten years. The aversions usually fade over time. Fortunately, I got over the aversion before I began to travel to the Far East.

These food aversions have been studied extensively in animals. They are unlike many other kinds of learned responses. An animal will associate a taste with an illness, even if the illness comes twelve hours later. These studies have also shown that the association is not a result of regurgitation from the illness. These aversions are powerful, and quite independent of conscious thought.

Because of the inability of conscious thought to control appetite, at least in most of us, reduced-calorie diets appear to have two effects that are likely to doom them as a strategy in weight loss. First, as I have mentioned before, appetite is increased and metabolism is slowed to defend the set point. Second, animal studies have shown that deprivation also alters the kind of foods that are preferred. Specifically, the preference for fat is increased. Although studies of extreme deprivation in humans are rare, they have been done. When food becomes available again, the person overeats and actually gains past the original pre-deprivation weight. As in the animal studies, the preference shifts toward foods high in fat and sugar.

Keeping in mind that the appetite-control mechanisms are not under conscious control, overeating and eating as much fat as possible are actually sensible biological strategies to adopt in the face of reduced availability of food. If the appetite mechanisms determine that food is scarce, it makes sense to eat as much as possible at the times that food is available, and to prefer fat since it packs in the most calories and sugar because it is the quickest way to make calories available to the metabolic system. The set-point mechanisms do not attempt to determine the cause of the food deprivation. They simply detect the change in body fat, weight, and food intake, and adjust the appetite and metabolism accordingly.

While we are on the topic of food deprivation, I should mention the effects of stress on appetite. The term "comfort food" has always had meaning to me. For me, it was pot roast or sausage and eggs. In my travels to the United Kingdom, I quickly discovered the "full English breakfast," with its eggs, sausage, fried potatoes, and toast. This is an institution of comfort food. It is very appealing when you are stressed out from travel. When I was traveling in Asia, all of the hotels that were frequented by westerners featured huge breakfast buffets which included all the components of the full English breakfast and much more. I found them very attractive under the stress of the very long trip, the strange (to me) environment, and the pressures of conducting business in a different culture.

It turns out that the concept of "comfort food" has currency in the scientific literature. Comfort food is food that is preferred under stress and which actually appears to reduce the stress. Comfort foods are dense in calories. In a recent study, adults were asked to recall their favorite comfort foods. The leading choices are listed in Table 3.1.

TABLE 3.1 • MOST POPULAR COMFORT FOODS			
FOOD	PERCENTAGE CHOOSING	FOOD	PERCENTAGE CHOOSING
Potato chips	23	Candy/chocolate	11%
Ice cream	14	Pasta or pizza	11%
Cookies	12	Steak or beef burgers	9%

This list is not good news for overweight individuals who are stressed. This is a particular problem when you consider that calorie restriction is itself a very stressful experience. Except for pasta, these are calorie-dense foods, and all are full of refined carbohydrates and/or saturated fat. Whether pasta is high fat and high calorie depends upon the sauce. Fettuccini Alfredo and spaghetti with meatballs definitely fit there. On the other hand, I have many recipes for pasta that are much healthier. (For some of these recipes, see Chapter 9.)

Animal studies confirm this idea of the influence of stress on food preferences. Rats subjected to chronic stress shift their preference away from rat chow toward sugar and lard. Again, we are seeing a preference of calorie-dense foods, in the form of either refined carbohydrates or saturated fat.

IF LOW-FAT DIETS AND LOW-CALORIE DIETS ARE NOT VERY EFFECTIVE, WHAT CAN YOU DO?

The evidence I have discussed indicates the following:

1. Diets high in saturated fat raise the set point and contribute to overweight and obesity.

2. Stress and food deprivation both increase the preference for a high-calorie, high-fat diet.

3. Low-fat diets and reduced-calorie diets appear to be minimally effective strategies for sustained weight loss.

4. A Mediterranean Diet appears to be more effective for weight loss than other approaches. It is more sustainable, and, unlike low-calorie and low-fat diets, it appears to be an effective strategy for individuals who have maintained weight loss after obesity.

CAN A MEDITERRANEAN DIET RESET YOUR WEIGHT THERMOSTAT?

I believe that a Mediterranean Diet does indeed enable you to reset your weight thermostat and lower your set point. To be sure, there is no direct evidence of this. All of the evidence is indirect. It includes:

1. Populations that eat the Mediterranean Diet have lower set points, that is, less obesity.

2. A Mediterranean Diet for weight loss is more sustainable than other approaches, indicating that they are better able to overcome the set-point mechanisms that defend body weight, even when the weight is too high.

3. In the extreme case, healthy eating, which is similar to the Mediterranean Diet, appears to be the most effective strategy for sustained weight loss in obese individuals. Low-calorie and low-fat diets are just as common in the groups that fail as in the group that succeeds in long-term weight loss.

Why might it be that the Mediterranean Diet would be more effective at lowering the set point than other approaches? For one thing it is a more natural approach. Trying to reduce calories is not only unpleasant, but it directly challenges the set-point mechanism. It activates the defense mechanisms of slower metabolism and increased appetite. This is like calisthenics for the set-point mechanism. The evidence suggests that the mechanism does not get fatigued in the face of the challenge of a low-calorie diet. What usually gets fatigued is our willpower to overcome our increased appetite.

The approach I describe in *The Laguna Beach Diet* does not focus on calories, but on eating the right foods. These are the foods that, if we had always eaten them, we would probably not have a weight problem. It is my belief that this diet provides a nutritional environment that, combined with exercise, enables the thermostat to move its set point to a much healthier weight level. Trying to force the set point down with low-fat, low-calorie diets creates huge resistance from the set-point mechanism. Switching to the diet I recommend does not mobilize the defensive strategies of the set-point mechanism.

In the remainder of the book, I will elaborate on the concepts and principles expressed in this chapter. The next chapter is a step-by-step guide to the process that my wife and I have used successfully. I will describe in detail a style of eating and activity that will enable you to lose weight and improve your health. I will explain how to make the transition from your present lifestyle to the new lifestyle. I will give you tools to stay on the right path if you have difficulty. Later chapters will provide more information on how what you eat affects your health, provide recipes for simple and delicious meals, and explain how to stay with the eating style when dining out or ordering in.

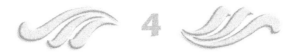

How to Find the Path and Stay on It

WHILE THE PROCESS THAT I RECOMMEND in *The Laguna Beach Diet* is relatively simple, be assured that it requires change. To paraphrase a line I heard many times as a business consultant, "if you always do what you always did, you'll always get what you always got." While the changes are not fighting against your biological set-point mechanism, they are dramatic changes nevertheless. The difficulty of change must not be underestimated.

STOPPING AND STARTING

It may sound simple, but if you intend to change what you are doing, you have to stop some of the things you are doing now. The hardest part of change is usually not the starting of new activities, but the stopping of old ones. Realize that this is especially true when we are talking about eating habits. The fundamental controls of eating are not in the rational part of the brain (the cerebral cortex) but in the more primitive, emotional parts of the brain (particularly the hypothalamus). Emotions are likely to arise as we attempt to change this behavior. Expect this. While the process that I recommend is easier than any other weight-loss system that I have found, it is by no means without its trials.

I quit smoking nearly forty years ago after two unsuccessful attempts each lasting six months. My third attempt was finally successful. This success was based, in part, on my understanding of the problems that arose when I tried to break the habit. First was the realization that simply changing a routine causes discomfort. If you are accustomed to answering the phone when it rings, you will experience a slight discomfort when you let it ring and do not answer. Avoiding a food that you are in the habit of eating and enjoy can cause a lot of discomfort. It is important to recognize this discomfort as a natural result of the change, and not a signal of some deep and meaningful need. You just have to live with it for a while. It will go away. However, some individuals cannot tolerate this discomfort and will be unable to make the changes required to follow the program that I am recommending.

The second key realization for me was that smoking was not one habit, but several. I smoked when I had my first cup of coffee in the morning. I smoked after finishing a meal, and so on. These habits were quickly broken as I encountered them on a daily basis. However, I also smoked at cocktail parties. Since I did not attend one until months after I quit smoking, that habit was not extinguished. At the first cocktail party I went to, I experienced a powerful rebirth of my craving for cigarettes. Had I not realized that this was a separate habit, I would have been very discouraged and concluded that the cravings would never go away and that I would eventually succumb to them and start smoking again. Realizing that this was just one of my last surviving smoking habits enabled me to get through the experience easily.

The last smoking habit I broke was smoking when I rode a motorcycle. Actually I would smoke when I stopped, since it is difficult (but possible) to smoke while riding. Just before I quit smoking I had sold my motorcycle and did not get another one for a long time. Twenty years later I bought one. I went for a ride, demounted, and experienced a craving that I had not felt in many years.

Your own eating habits are likely to be multiple. For example, if you usually eat steak when dining out in a fine restaurant, you will experience that craving the first few times you go to a fine restaurant. Another example of particular food habits is the concept of comfort food, which I discussed in the previous chapter. It is something you might look forward to after a hard week, or while eating alone on a business trip. While each person has his or her own choice of comfort food, most of the foods in this category have a very high fat and/or sugar content. I mentioned that for my wife and me, comfort food meant some form of beef. Since we have been in this process of change, it has switched to pasta, but not without some emotional struggle, especially for my wife. I think that existing habits regarding comfort food may be the biggest problem with the change I am recommending. Because the change itself is stressful, it may evoke the desire for comfort food. Avoiding your old comfort food can increase the stress.

The point of all this is that you should not get discouraged when there is a bump in the road. Over time, the road will get smoother and smoother. That is the beauty of this particular process. With many other diets, the road will never get smooth, since you are fighting against your own set-point mechanisms, and severely limiting basic things like fats or carbohydrates, or even calories.

The following system of what to stop and what to start is an attempt to be realistic about the changes that will be required to succeed on this diet. It is more a set of principles than a map. You should review it to be sure that you can commit to following it.

Some years ago, I had an ongoing discussion with Dr. W. Edwards Deming about the nature of change. Dr. Deming was the brilliant teacher mentioned earlier who revolutionized industrial management in Japan, and did much to change business in the United States as well. He believed that change, like changing the way you manage or changing the way you eat, is a discontinuous process that happens all at once. It happens with a true commitment to change.

Because of my experience with 12-step programs, I believed that change was continuous, and happened gradually over time. According to Alcoholics Anonymous, you stay sober "one day at a time." You have never completed the change. You are always a "recovering alcoholic."

I currently believe that change is both continuous and discontinuous. First, there must be a commitment. That is a discontinuous step. However, the job is not complete. You must have the discipline to stay with the program. I have seen alcoholics and addicts relapse after as much as ten years of sobriety.

I would differ from traditional 12-step approaches in the severity that lapses are dealt with. Injecting heroin or sniffing cocaine is a very serious matter. Eating a steak is not. Eating steak frequently, however, will defeat the program. It is better to eat an occasional steak than to quit the program. With drug and alcohol addiction, the conventional wisdom is that you have to abstain forever. The list below is built in such a way as to deal with the problems that may arise at times when the process seems difficult. It contains escape hatches.

1. **Stop letting yourself get hungry.** There are two fundamental enemies of attempting to lose weight: hunger and animal fat. Hunger initiates a number of mechanisms that interfere with losing weight. Among these is the slowing of metabolism. In earlier times, extreme hunger was usually the result of a scarcity of food. (No evidence has yet been found of Jenny Craig-type programs to help the Neanderthals lose weight.) When food is scarce it makes biological sense to conserve it. Consequently, it is logical that when you are hungry, your metabolism slows to conserve energy. If you have lost weight through deprivation, this slowing of your metabolism ensures that you will have to eat even less to maintain the level you have achieved. Your set-point mechanism does not know *why* you are hungry.

   Sustained hunger is like putting your hunger drive on steroids. Hunger can become a very strong drive. In the long term, millions of dieters have learned that hunger is very likely to defeat willpower. Consider that this has an evolutionary benefit as well. If one gets distracted and skips a few meals, the drive to eat gets very strong. No matter how captivating the distraction, survival demands that you avoid starvation. Not only does the hunger drive increase, but also the appetite shifts in the direction of calorie-dense foods like sugar and fat. Although reports of fasting suggest that the drive can be overcome by some people, a direct confrontation with this drive is a poor approach for most of us. Certainly all of my attempts to lose weight through deprivation were unsuccessful because my hunger drive proved in the end to be stronger than my willpower.

   The bottom line is that you should eat enough at a meal to feel satisfied. If you get hungry, eat a healthy snack (See item 9 on page 57.)

2. **Conversely, stop eating when you are not hungry.** I have always been

frustrated and even angry at parents who insist that their child eat at mealtime and eat all that they are served. They even offer praise for eating. Eating should be controlled by appetite, not by attempting to please one's parent. You should not train your child to eat when he or she is not hungry. Assuming that the child does not have a serious neurological or psychiatric disorder, the child's appetite-control mechanisms will ensure adequate nutrition.

I recall a story from graduate school that emphasizes the importance of appetite control, albeit in a somewhat different context. A very young child had an unusual hunger for salt. The parents were concerned about this and went to their family doctor. He told them that they should limit the child's salt intake, which they did. The child died. It turned out that the child had a kidney disorder and was losing too much salt in his urine. The appetite for salt was able to compensate for this until the family intervened at the advice of the physician.

The point of this last account is not that everyone should eat a lot of salt, but that specific hungers are often based on real needs and should not be dismissed as an aberration. If you are hungry, your brain is telling you that you need to eat. If you are not hungry, it is telling you that *you do not need to eat.*

3. **Stop worrying about calories.** Instead, worry about eating the wrong foods. This is a corollary of the avoidance of hunger. Your control system will induce you to eat enough calories in any day to satisfy its set point. If you do not get enough calories, you will be hungry, which is bad. Your goal is to satisfy your caloric requirements with the "right" foods, so that your set point will come down over time.

4. **Stop using red meat as a main source of protein.** You should eat very little red meat, but you can eat some. My own experience is the less red meat you eat, the less you want. I grew up in Kansas and was raised on Kansas City steak, which I loved. There are many very simple ways to make a delicious meal with beef. I had to change. I currently eat a small amount of red meat once or twice each month. Red meat appears to be a major culprit in setting our weight thermostat at too high a level. Staying away from it at the start may be a bit difficult, but is worth the

effort. My wife initially had a lot of trouble with this, but after being on diet for a number of months, her tastes changed, and she is now very happy with a diet in which most of the animal protein is poultry or seafood. She does eat an occasional, great, expensive, bun-less hamburger.

Instead of relying primarily on red meat for protein, we enjoy a greater variety. We eat one or two eggs each week. In many dishes I use ground turkey as a substitute for red meat because it has about half the saturated fat content. We also get protein from plant sources including legumes and soy. We frequently eat rice and beans, which is a source of complete protein. I often add a bit of meat in cooking the beans, to improve their flavor.

5. **Stop eating trans fat** (often listed on food labels as partially hydrogenated oils). Trans fat is an exceptionally effective builder of the arterial plaque that is an important component of coronary heart disease. It is even worse for you than the saturated fats found in red meat and dairy products. Trans fats are used to preserve the shelf-life of many processed foods like cakes, cookies, crackers, chips, and most margarines. As a general rule, you are much better off eating butter than eating margarine with trans fat. However, some new margarines, like Smart Balance, are made without trans fat.

6. **Stop believing that you need to eat dairy products.** According to an extensive review of the subject, "The data to support a public health recommendation about dairy food consumption are quite inconsistent, and any such recommendation is controversial." This does not mean that you should avoid dairy products altogether, just that they are not essential. For example, low-fat yogurt is good as a snack and as an ingredient in soups and sauces, but you should limit your intake of high-fat dairy products like butter, cream, whole milk, and fatty cheeses like cheddar. Parmesan grated over pasta is fine because the amount of cheese is so small. Feta crumbled over salad is fine. I use part-skim ricotta in lasagna, and sometimes use goat milk cheeses for their lower fat content.

There is no reason to drink milk to maintain health. It turns out that you really *do* outgrow your need for milk. While butter has a distinctive taste in cooking, I generally substitute olive oil. For spreading on toast, Smart Balance margarine, which contains a blend of soy, palm, canola, and olive oils, and no trans fat, is okay, as is peanut butter if it is not hydrogenated or sweetened. Even better is the use of avocado or hummus (a spread made from chickpeas and sesame seeds). Hummus is easy to make, and very nutritious.

7. **Stop eating most processed foods.** Although you can find some processed foods that are healthy, most contain too much salt, the wrong kinds of fat, unhealthy sugars, and refined carbohydrates.

8. **Stop avoiding oils and carbohydrates.** Many people who have a weight problem feel that they must continue to avoid oils and carbohydrates when they go on a Mediterranean Diet. Olive oil is a critical component of this diet. Unlike some other diets, which attempt to limit fat to as low as 15 percent of total calories, the Mediterranean Diet includes about 35 percent of total calories as fat. Olive oil is especially important, and you should make sure you get enough. What you should avoid is *saturated* fats, like the fat found in dairy products and red meat. To be sure, fish and poultry also contain saturated fat, but they contain much less.

   Many people resist Mediterranean-style diets because these diets rely on carbohydrates. This resistance is based on the mistaken belief that carbohydrates themselves will cause you to gain weight. However, it is the combination of refined carbohydrates and high levels of saturated fat that cause you to gain weight. Carbohydrate-rich foods such as grains, fruits, and vegetables are fundamental to our diet. Since saturated fat is limited on this diet, the carbohydrates help you lose weight, not gain it.

9. **Start having healthy snacks on hand such as whole-grain bread, nuts, and fruit to deal with hunger.** Since you do not want to be hungry, you need something to stave it off until the next meal. The worst thing you can do is to eat processed foods like cookies and cakes. I rarely eat pastry, although a small portion once or twice a week is okay (if you do this, avoid trans fat). I use cashew nuts, apples, and bread with peanut

butter. While the nuts and peanut butter are high in fat, they are basic foods of the Mediterranean Diet. I have lost weight and maintained the loss while snacking on these foods. Any variety of nuts is okay, including nut butters, if they are not sweetened or hydrogenated (which is often done to prevent oil separation). Any fresh fruit is okay. I do allow myself a few squares of a semi-sweet chocolate bar (I prefer Lindt) as often as once each day. The longer I am with the diet, the less frequently I want this.

Mireille Guiliano, author of *French Women Don't Get Fat* (Knopf, 2004), recommends homemade yogurt for snacks, which is fine. If you use store-bought yogurt, use a low-fat or non-fat version with no sugar added. Whatever is available for a snack is okay if it fits the diet. Many processed snack foods do not.

10. **Start exercising moderately for at least thirty minutes, four times per week.** Exercise is an important mechanism for adjusting the setting of the weight-control thermostat. However, you do not have to become a marathon runner or tri-athlete. While more exercise is better, it is not that much better. Four sessions of thirty minutes of brisk walking each week will support the Mediterranean Diet regimen and enable weight loss. I believe that this is near the minimum, but it is quite sufficient. It is good that this is not a terribly ambitious regimen. It means you can achieve it and stay with it. Do more if you want, but do not do less.

As with any exercise program, you should consult with your physician to make sure that this will be safe for you.

11. **Start eating fresh fruits and fresh vegetables, whole-grains, whole-grain breads, and beans.** The food companies will not like this recommendation, but it is the only way to go. Frozen vegetables are okay but not as tasty as fresh, and far less flexible in what you can do with them. Do not use quick-cooking rice. Get a rice cooker. You put in the rice and the water, turn it on, and dish it out about forty-five minutes later.

It is not always easy to find good whole-grain breads. Many breads advertised as whole grain or whole wheat have some whole-grain flour, but a lot of refined flour. Also, in my experience, a lot of the whole-grain breads contain too much honey or sugar. Apparently, the bakers assume that we will not really like whole-grain bread. If you do buy bread made with honey or sugar, make sure that it is very low on the ingredients list. You might consider a bread machine. There are several good ones on the market, and whole-grain flour is widely available. Besides whole wheat, you may want to try using amaranth, buckwheat, cornmeal, rye, triticale, teff, spelt, and other whole-grain flours.

I rarely eat any canned beans or vegetables. Not only is their taste inferior, but they also usually have a high-sodium content and a variety of other additives. For example, I always cook beans from dried beans. The only exception is garbanzos. Cooking dried beans is a bit of a pain for someone who is pressed for time. One way to short cut the preparation time for dried beans is to use a pressure cooker. (See the section on Equipment on page 136 for more details.)

Fresh fruit is critical. If you are not snacking on fruit (see item 9 on page 57), add it for breakfast or dessert. I usually eat an apple each day for breakfast. It makes the most sense to eat what is in season when you can.

12. **Start favoring Italian, Asian, and Middle Eastern restaurants.** As the lifestyle of Americans has changed, dining out has become much more frequent, especially among the groups that will most likely read this book. From 1995 through 2004, the U.S. Department of Agriculture (USDA) reports that about 46 percent of consumer food expenditures were made for meals away from home. Their explanation is the obvious one. Many households are two-job families. Time for cooking and dishwashing are scarce. Most alarming is the fact that fast-food restaurants account for nearly 40 percent of this expenditure. Because they are cheaper, they likely account for more than 50 percent of meals eaten away from home.

Dining out is a fact of life for most of us, just like more expensive gasoline. You will have to learn to cope with it. For most of us, it means changing the restaurants we frequent and changing the menu items we select. If you are careful you can maintain this program and have excellent meals, albeit with a higher cost than home-cooked food. The easiest restaurants for me to find the right food are Italian,

Middle Eastern, seafood, Vietnamese, and Japanese. Chapter 7 focus-es on how to select healthy restaurants and healthy offerings.

13. **Start weighing yourself frequently, but do not get caught up in daily fluctuations.** My weight may go up or down as much as 3 pounds from day to day. Look for the trend over a thirty-day period. Apparently, many people who successfully lose weight get on the scale daily. I weigh myself four to five times per week. The best way to see how you are doing is to plot the weights on a chart, where the x-axis (horizontal) is days and the y-axis (vertical) is your weight. This will enable you to seen the trend. Chapter 5 will provide more detail on this.

    Weight loss is not precipitous with this diet. You should expect to lose in the range of 2 to 5 pounds per month from the start. If you are losing much more than that, you may be eating too little. What you are looking for is a sustained and substantial loss, not an instant fit into the clothes you wore five years ago.

14. **Stop being rigid about your diet.** It is better to indulge occasionally, rather than go off the diet. At first, for example, you may miss the red meat. I think that this is more of a habit than a specific hunger. After a few months that hunger abates. Steak still tastes good, but you will probably not have a craving for it. If you do have a strong craving, you are better off giving in to it from time to time rather than deciding that you cannot stay with the diet.

    My wife and I love to drive to Ensenada, in Mexico, for a two- or three-day holiday. The drive is only about two hours from our house and the contrast with San Diego is extreme. However, some Mexican food is nearly the opposite of the Mediterranean Diet. One of our favorite restaurants there is called Guadalajara. It is a plain restaurant that is very popular with the locals, but sees few tourists. The menu consists of *carne asada,* which is steak, marinated and then grilled over charcoal. After grilling, the steak is cut into strips and served with their fresh tortillas, rice, and beans. We always eat there when we go, in spite of our general avoidance of red meat. We view this as an infrequent indulgence, not as dropping out of the program.

    When I was well along with this book, my wife made a very funny confession to me. Early on in her weight-loss process, she had an irresistible craving for a hamburger. She got in her car and went to the drive-thru at the local Jack-in-the-Box. She ordered a sourdough Jack and ate it in the car in the empty parking lot behind the grocery store. Fran has been extremely successful in losing weight, allowing us frequent laughs about the guilt that surrounded her transgression. The moral, of course, is that you do not have to be perfect to be perfectly wonderful.

15. **Give yourself at least sixty days to adjust to the diet.** If you are not enjoying it, feeling better, and losing weight, either you are doing something wrong, or this diet is not for you. This is a lifestyle change, not a short-term diet to get your weight down. You will eventually reach a plateau. I went from 198 to about 182 in six months and stayed at that weight for more than one year. Then I began to lose weight again, reaching 173 a year later. I am happy with the current weight and feel good. If I wanted to lose more, I would probably need to increase my exercise.

It is critical that you not feel chronically hungry or deprived. If you do, you need to adjust. Remember, you are not trying to avoid calories. You are trying to eat the right foods. If you feel hungry or deprived, the process will not work.

WHAT SHOULD YOU ACTUALLY EAT?

In this next section, I will explain what my wife and I actually eat on a daily basis. This is done as an illustration. As long as you stay within the guidelines of the diet, summarized in the inset on pages 62–63, you can eat what *you* like, rather than conforming to what *we* like.

I enjoy eating. I do not enjoy the preparation of elaborate and complex dishes. I like relatively simple food, prepared from excellent ingredients. More important, I like it cooked to my taste. Anthony Bourdain, a successful New York chef and author of the wonderful book, *Kitchen Confidential* (Bloomsbury, 2000), writes that he loves to be invited out for dinner. Restaurants prepare standardized food designed to please their average patron. Home-cooked meals, prepared by a competent cook, are more interesting and often much better.

I am a competent cook, or at worst I have been fortunate enough to have had very polite dinner guests over the years. I am not a chef, nor do I ever intend to be. A chef is competent to prepare consistent food for many people in an efficient and economical manner. I am not interested in stan-

MY LAGUNA BEACH DIET

- **Beans:** All varieties, including black, cranberry, garbanzo, lentils, limas, pinto, red, split peas, soy, and others. (Avoid using canned beans that contain salt and additives.)

- **Beverages:** Water, fruit juices and vegetable juices (if minimally processed, without sweeteners), tea, coffee, and wine (one to three glasses a day, as long as you do not have other health or behavioral concerns that argue against this).

- **Dairy products:** One percent and low-fat milk, yogurt (unsweetened), and cottage cheese; part-skim ricotta and mozzarella; goat cheese. Use small quantities of higher fat cheeses such as Parmesan, Romano, feta, Fontina, Monterey Jack, cheddar, and Swiss, for garnish. (Restrict meals with lots of cheese, like macaroni and cheese—which I really like—to two times per month.)

- **Eggs:** Boiled, poached, or scrambled or fried in olive or canola oil. (Limit to four weekly.)

- **Fish and seafood:** All fresh and saltwater varieties grilled, poached, baked, pan-roasted, or sautéed in olive oil.

- **Fruits:** All varieties at least three a day. (Avoid canned, bottled, or frozen fruits with sweeteners added.)

- **Grains:** All whole grains (brown rice, oats, barley, millet, couscous, bulgur, quinoa, etc.) and products such as breads, cereals, crackers, and pasta containing minimally processed whole grains.

dardization and my cooking declines when the guest list exceeds six to eight persons. My dishes are designed around what I like, what ingredients are available, cost, and what I happen to have in stock from previous meals. If I go to buy fish, I buy what is fresh, not something I planned for dinner. The recipe should fit the ingredients as much as the ingredients should fit the recipe.

- **Meats:** Favor skinless turkey and chicken. Use red meats as flavoring. (Limit red meat meals to a 4-ounce portion about twice a month and avoid luncheon meats such as salami, bologna, liverwurst, and other processed meats that are high in saturated fat, sodium, and other chemicals.)

- **Nuts and seeds:** All varieties, including nut and seed butters like almond, macadamia, pumpkin, sunflower, tahini (sesame seed butter), and walnut.

- **Oils (fats):** Cold-pressed extra-virgin olive oil, canola oil (for a milder flavor for cooking), butter-like spreads such as Smart Balance, or butter used sparingly. (Avoid saturated fats, hydrogenated margarines, and products containing trans fats.)

- **Seasonings and condiments:** All herbs and spices; use mayonnaise (made with olive or canola oil), sweetened ketchup, and other condiments sparingly.

- **Soups and stews:** All bean-, rice-, and vegetable-based with chicken, fish, or small amounts of beef, pork, or lamb added. (Avoid cream-based and canned soups with salt and additives.)

- **Sweets:** All fresh, frozen, stewed, canned, and bottled fruits (without sweeteners); small amounts of chocolate. (Limit pastries such as cookies, pies, and cakes to small portions once or twice a week.)

- **Vegetables:** All varieties, at least two servings a day, raw, baked, lightly steamed, or sautéed or braised in olive or canola oil.

This last point is illustrated by a story I heard several years ago. There is a farm in Rancho Santa Fe, an elite suburb of San Diego. It is about four miles from my home. The farm is run by the Chinos, a family of Japanese descent. It sits on tens of millions of dollars worth of real estate, but the Chinos are committed to farming. They produce vegetables and fruits of incomparable quality. Years ago, they were discovered by Alice Waters, owner of Chez Panisse restaurant and the inventor of California cuisine, and by Wolfgang Puck. Both had standing orders with the farm, but nothing was specified. Each day the farm would pack up what was the best produce they had that day and put it on a bus for the Bay Area. Puck and Waters built their menus around the ingredients rather than building the ingredients around the menu.

To cook the way I do takes some experience. You need to learn what tastes good to you, what ingredients work well together, and what types of preparation will give you the result you want. Formal instruction can help, but will not substitute for practice.

A huge advantage of learning to cook this way is that you can then take dishes that you like and adapt them to the Laguna Beach Diet's Mediterranean-style of eating. So far, I have done a good job with chili and meatloaf. It took much longer to perfect turkey burgers, but now we are happy with them. Of course, there is always the possibility that we just gave up our quest for the perfect turkey burger, and decided to accept what we had. The recipe is in Chapter 9, so you can see for yourself.

Understanding a bit about cooking is important in another respect. I expect that a substantial proportion of the readers of this book eat many of their meals in restaurants. Having an idea of how food is prepared will enable you to make choices that are a better fit for a Mediterranean-style diet. For example, I can make excellent and healthy mashed potatoes using olive oil and herbs. However, they are usually prepared with butter and often with cream and are therefore not a good choice in restaurants.

Chapter 9 provides many recipes for the Laguna Beach Diet. Any cookbook can provide many more. The Internet is probably the best reference source. I frequently use the search engine on the Food Network site (www.foodnetwork.com). Many of the recipes there are from distinguished sources, and are evaluated in terms of time, difficulty, and satisfaction.

I rarely follow one of these very closely. If I want to make a new dish, I will look at a number of recipes and then decide how to make the dish, based on what ingredients I have, simplicity, and the expected taste. Usually, it is a synthesis of several recipes plus my own modifications.

The breakfast, lunch, and dinner choices below represent what my wife and I eat. They will work for what you cook and they will also serve as a guide for ordering in a restaurant (discussed in detail in Chapter 7). I have listed categories here, not individual dishes.

Breakfast

- Fresh fruit: All varieties are okay.

- Oatmeal: Preferably steel-cut (not instant or rolled) oats with 1 percent fat milk.

- Dry cereals: Made from whole grains with no sweeteners added with 1 percent fat milk.

- Eggs: Occasionally (no more than four eggs per week), and cooked in olive or canola oil, not butter.

- Toast: Whole-grain bread with olive oil, Smart Balance margarine, nut butters (no hydrogenated oils or added sugar), or hummus.

- Beverages: Tea, especially green tea, or coffee.

Lunch

I usually eat leftovers from dinner because I work from home. Basically, any dinner menu is okay for lunch. Usually the portions are smaller and there are fewer courses. I rarely prepare anything like this just for lunch, as I do not want to spend that much time. If we do not have dinner leftovers, I usually make a sandwich.

- Sandwiches: I often use sardines (when my wife is not home because she thinks they are gross). Also I eat tuna salad, sliced chicken, or turkey, all without mayonnaise. Cheese sandwiches have quite a bit of saturated fat, so I do not recommend them, nor do I recommend luncheon meats (see

Meats on page 63). When I am in a hurry I eat a piece of whole-grain toast with peanut butter (without sugar or trans fat). I actually like it with mustard but sliced bananas are more popular.

- Tacos: Chicken or fish tacos are okay. Use leftover chicken or fish. Burritos are not as good, because most brands of flour tortillas are made with shortening. Our local organic market sells chicken and veggie burritos in a whole-wheat tortilla. These are all right, though they are certainly not thrilling. In general, I do not like the whole-wheat tortillas nearly as much as I like the corn.

Snack Foods

- Bread (whole grain) plain, with olive oil, Smart Balance, or peanut butter
- Cereal (whole grain, no sugar)
- Cottage cheese (low fat)
- Fruit
- Nuts and seeds
- Raw vegetables with or without a dip made from low-fat yogurt
- Rice cakes and other types of whole-grain crackers
- Yogurt (low fat, no sugar)

Dinner

Main Courses

- Chicken dishes: The healthiest choice is boneless, skinless breast, which contains the least saturated fat. I usually marinate these and pan-roast them.

- Fish and seafood dishes: Grilled, pan-roasted, poached, baked, or steamed. Use olive or canola oil for pan-roasting.

- Pasta dishes: Countless varieties. I use commercial pasta, often the whole-wheat variety, or fresh pasta made locally. Our favorite sauces include a fish sauce, a sauce based on garbanzo beans, and the old stand-by, Bolognese (with a ground turkey instead of beef). Avoid cream sauces and eat the Bolognese only occasionally. (You'll find the recipes for several sauces in Chapter 9.)

- Soups and stews: Countless homemade varieties using vegetables, beans, chicken or fish, or small amounts of beef, pork, or lamb. Again, avoid cream and canned soups.

- Turkey dishes, turkey meatloaf, and turkey burgers: Ground turkey has about 60 percent as much saturated fat as 90 percent lean ground beef. (See Table 1.1, "Saturated Fat Information for Some Common Foods" on page 19.) Ground turkey breast, available in some stores, has much less than that. I often use a mixture of breast and dark-meat turkey, as the ground breast is a bit bland.

- Rice and bean dishes: All varieties.

- Chef's salad: This is an excuse to use up all sorts of leftovers. We include meats and cheeses in small quantities. Make the salad dressing with olive oil and vinegar or lemon. Avoid prepared salad dressings as they often contain trans fat and considerable quantities of sodium.

Side Dishes

- Beans: All varieties of dried beans, fresh beans, and frozen beans.

- Broccoli: Steamed lightly or sautéed.

- Brown rice (steamed): As I mentioned earlier in the chapter, get a rice cooker. I sometimes add vegetables like peas, sautéed mushrooms, or sautéed chunks of eggplant to the rice after it is steamed.

- Cauliflower: Baked, lightly steamed, stir-fried, or mashed like mashed potatoes. This is a bit healthier than potatoes, if you have a taste for it. I hated it but cooked it because my wife loved it. Now I like it too.

- Dark leafy greens: Collard greens, dandelion greens, kale, rapini, spinach, and Swiss chard, steamed lightly, sautéed, or braised.

- Eggplant: Usually roasted, grilled, or sautéed in olive oil.

- Potatoes: Baked, boiled, mashed (with low-fat milk and olive oil) or stir-fried in olive or canola oil.

- Squash: All varieties baked, lightly steamed, or stir-fried.

- Sweet potatoes, yams: If you can get really good ones, you can just bake them and eat them with nothing on them but a little salt.

- Salad: All varieties of lettuce and fresh vegetables. Make the salad dressing with olive oil and vinegar or lemon.

THE BOTTOM LINE

The approach I have described here has worked for us. It is based on a great deal of scientific research. This approach avoids the discomfort of hunger and radical measures like the avoidance of fat or carbohydrates. It does require a significant reduction, for most of us, in the consumption of saturated fats and refined carbohydrates. But it is really an approach of adding rather than subtracting. You increase your consumption of olive oil, fish, poultry, fresh fruits and vegetables, whole grains, legumes, nuts and seeds, and red wine. Chapter 5 has a scientific scale to measure your adherence to the Laguna Beach Diet. Of the fourteen questions in this scale, ten are oriented toward consumption and only four are about avoidance.

The approach may require some changes in your selection of recipes and menus for cooking, and your choice of restaurants and menu selections when dining out, but it will not require you to sacrifice quality or enjoyment in eating. That is an important reason that this is a sustainable approach. If you are on a diet, you need to ask yourself if you would like to eat this way for the rest of your life. If the answer is "no," then you are on the wrong diet.

EXERCISE AND CALORIES

An hour of jogging will burn about 600 calories, while an hour of walking, about 300. One pound of fat equals about 3,500 calories. Therefore, six hours of jogging in a week might burn off one pound, all other things being equal, which they are probably not.

THE ROLE OF EXERCISE

Exercise burns calories. However, it is not clear that exercise, in itself, is a way to lose weight. Although it seems logical that when we use up calories in exercise, our regulatory system would detect that and we would eat more to compensate. There is a lot of scientific research on this topic, and it turns out that this is generally not true. Though this would then suggest that exercise would be a good way to lose weight, this turns out to not be true either, at least for moderate levels of exercise. First, it takes a lot of exercise to lose significant weight (see the inset "Exercise and Calories"). Second, when fat declines, the set-point mechanisms should detect the loss of fat and weight and attempt to increase appetite and decrease metabolism to get back to the original setting.

However, it appears that exercise is an essential *component* of an effective weight-loss program. Jean Mayer, the famous nutrition scientist, proposed years ago that a moderate level of exercise is necessary for the set-point mechanism to function properly. In both animal and human studies, Mayer showed that strongly reducing activity levels led to overweight and obesity. Subsequent research has supported Mayer's observations.

Our experience is that the combination of the Laguna Beach Diet with moderate exercise, at least thirty minutes four times each week, enables the resetting of one's weight thermostat to a healthier level. It is not just the fact that the exercise is burning calories, but that it is enabling the set-point mechanism to function properly. My own experience indicates that both diet and exercise are necessary. I was overweight before I adopted this diet, even though I exercised more than I do now.

In reviewing this diet and exercise regimen, there is nothing on it that requires strong discipline or that causes significant discomfort. Sure there are some days that I do not feel like going for a thirty to forty-five minute walk, but that is a very minor problem. My own life is much better. I feel better when I wake up. I have more energy during the day, and I sleep better at night. The food is great, and there is plenty of it. For my wife and me, it is a way of life.

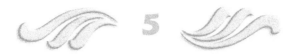

5

Monitoring Your Progress

THIS CHAPTER WAS WRITTEN in cooperation with my friend Pat Ragan. Pat is Vice President for Quality, Safety, Health, and Environment at Bayer CropScience. As a consultant, I have worked with Pat for more than ten years. We have become a team, using measurement methods I learned and used as a scientist to solve business problems, and have written a book together on measurement in business. Among the many things Pat brings to the table is his business experience. This ensures that our processes are practical. His counsel in this area is invaluable.

Ultimately, the assessment of how well you are doing would include measures like weight, your waist circumference, your blood lipids (total cholesterol, ratio of HDL to LDL, triglycerides, etc.), your blood pressure, and insulin sensitivity (which relates to whether you are at risk of developing type 2 diabetes).

CHARTING YOUR WEIGHT—A BETTER *WEIGH*

Some say that you should rarely weigh yourself if you are in a weight-loss process. I believe that the hypothesis here is that weighing yourself is stressful. However, the data I have seen indicates that successful weight losers weigh themselves more frequently than unsuccessful ones. Whether this frequent weighing is a cause of successful weight loss is not proven by such data, however. It may be that it is a result, not a cause. Perhaps successful weight losers enjoy the results of weight measurement more than unsuccessful ones, so they do it more often. Nevertheless, as a scientist and a businessman, I am firmly of the belief that if you want to change something, you should measure it. Therefore, I strongly recommend weighing yourself several times each week. My wife and I have done this throughout our process, and continue to do it today.

It is also useful to measure the other important parameters mentioned above, and have the results reviewed by your physician. Measures of cholesterol and blood pressure should be taken, along with some measure that indicates whether you are on the way to developing a diabetic condition. This can be done at your annual physical, or more or less frequently according to your physician's direction.

Before you start measuring however, there are some things you need to consider. For example, all measures vary. Even if your weight is not changing, you will not weigh the same every day. To reduce variation, you should weigh yourself with no clothing, and at about the same time of day. You typically weigh the least first thing in the morning, unless you engage in strenuous exercise during the day. If you weigh in the morning, try to do so before having breakfast and it will improve the consistency of the result. Still, there will be some variation. Some days you may have a bit more fluid on board. Some days you may have more contents in your intestines. I am sure there are more sources of variation, but I expect these are the greatest sources. With my weight tracking steadily at an average of 183, it would go as low as 180 and as high as 185. The more you weigh

MAKE SURE THERE IS A TREND BEFORE YOU TRY TO RESPOND

It is important that you avoid responding to random fluctuations. If you deprive yourself after an unusually heavy day and allow yourself to go off the diet and indulge a bit after an unusually lean day, the process will not work as well. In the language of quality control theory, this is called "over-adjustment." It will increase variation in the process, and interfere with the ability to get a consistent outcome. The proper basis for revising the process is the discovery of a real trend, or lack of one.

the wider this variation will be. A 5-pound swing is not unusual for someone over 200 pounds.

The reason to chart your weight is to be able to differentiate between this random variation and actual changes in your weight. There is an elegant and important statistical methodology to accomplish this, but it is not really necessary for you to do something so complicated. The measurement itself is important. What you are really measuring are the effects of the changes you are making. You want to know what works and does not work for *you.*

It is very important to know what works on a long-term basis and what gives only short-term results that cannot be sustained. My friend Pat relays the experience of high school, when he practiced football on hot August days. He would lose as much as 10 pounds in a $2\frac{1}{2}$ hour session. Almost all would have returned by the next day because it was nearly all water loss. With proper tracking of your eating habits, lifestyle, and your weight, you can distinguish the sustained changes from the temporary fluctuations. If you are like my wife and me, you will begin to feel enthusiastic about your progress. This enthusiasm will reinforce the changes you are making.

Weigh yourself at least three times each week and plot your weight on a chart like the one in Figure 3 on page 74. Many people like to track their weight on a computer, but my experience is that a simple piece of graph paper near your scale will work best. If I were to use my laptop in the relatively tight space of my bathroom, I would probably drop it into the bathtub. Don't make the collection of this information too complex or it will not get done. You can enter the data in you computer later (in a different room) but the act of placing the point on the paper and watching the line is a powerful reminder of the change you are trying to make and how well you are doing. This chart represents one month of daily weighings.

There is a trend of weight loss here. The average weight in the first week is 189.7 and 184.4 the last week. I arrived at this number simply by taking an average of points in the first week and taking an average of the points in the last week. In fact, looking at the average for the first week of a month and comparing it with the average for the last week is a simple way to see the trend. A statistician (like me) would look at this and note that every point in the last week is lower than any point in the first week, providing

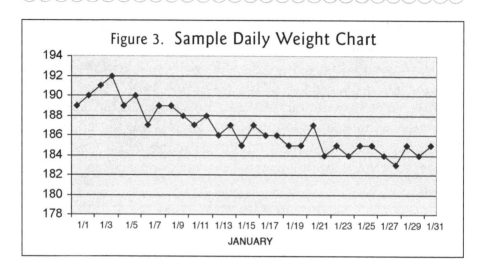

Figure 3. Sample Daily Weight Chart

statistical assurance that the trend is real. If the last week of the month is about the same or higher than the first week, your weight management efforts may not be working. If the last week of the second month is about the same as the first week of the preceding month, you are not yet losing weight, and you need to do some troubleshooting, which is discussed later in the chapter.

Of course, even if you are very successful at losing weight, you will eventually come to a point where your weight is stable. It may be more than you would really like, or it may not, but you cannot keep losing indefinitely. Your weight thermostat will always have a set point. Your objective is to achieve a set point that keeps you healthy and lets you feel good about yourself. If you want to be a runway model, a cyclist in the Tour de France, or a sumo wrestler, you will need a personal trainer, a lot of work, the right genes, and a different book.

Perhaps the most important point to be made here relates to the first week. Many people would be concerned at seeing their weight go from 189 to 192. Worse, they might try to do something about it. This would be a serious mistake. They would be responding to random variation, and most likely interfering with the process. To establish a real trend in a short period requires seven consecutive points each above the previous average. It is critical to ignore the random variation and attend only to the longer-term trends.

ASSESSING YOUR ADHERENCE TO THE PROCESS

Measures like weight, cholesterol levels, and insulin sensitivity are what are called "end of process measures." They reflect the results of prior actions. Sometimes, the actions may have occurred days, weeks, or even months before. Therefore, it is also important to have what is referred to as "in process measures." They tell us if our process is being carried out properly early in the game.

A number of researchers have developed questionnaires to evaluate adherence to a Mediterranean Diet. Most of these are quite long and tedious, but recently some shorter scales have been developed and validated. The one below is derived from a scale developed by a Spanish group under the leadership of Dr. Miguel Martinez-Gonzales. What "validation" means is that a statistical study has been carried out, demonstrating that people with higher scores are less likely to have cardiovascular disease. It is a reasonable assumption that higher scores will also lead to healthier weight.

When you are a month into the process, go ahead and score yourself. Our answer scores follow in italics.

1. Do you use olive oil as the principal fat for your cooking? Yes = 1 point. (*Yes, we rarely use any other oil.*)

2. How much olive oil do you consume each day (including what you use for cooking, salad dressings, etc.)? Two or more tablespoons = 1 point. (*We consume more than two tablespoons.*)

WHAT IS "VALIDATION"?

When you hear that a questionnaire has been *validated*, it has a technical meaning. It means that the score on the scale correlates with some other criterion measurement. IQ scales were originally validated against school achievement and economic success. Students with higher IQ scores got better grades and eventually made more money. People with higher scores on the Mediterranean-diet scale have less heart disease.

3. How many helpings of vegetables (including greens) do you eat each day? Two or more = 1 point. (*We eat more than two helpings.*)

4. How many pieces of fruit, including natural fruit juice, do you eat each day? Three or more = 1 point. (*Two to three pieces per day. We fall short here.*)

5. How many portions of red meat do you eat each day? (A portion is 4 to 5 ounces). Less than one portion each day = 1 point. (*We eat almost no red meat.*)

6. How many portions of butter, margarine, or cream do you consume each day (including use in cooking and sauces)? (A portion is 2 teaspoons.) No more than one each day = 1 point. (*We eat almost no butter, margarine, or cream.*)

7. How many sugar-sweetened beverages (soda, juice, etc.) do you drink each day? No more than one each day = 1 point. (*We drink none of these.*)

8. How much wine do you drink each week? Three or more glasses = 1 point. (*We drink about two glasses per day.*)

9. How many portions of legumes (beans, peas, lentils) do you eat each week? (A portion is 5 ounces.) Three or more each week = 1 point. (*We eat about three portions.*)

10. How many portions of fish or seafood do you eat each week? A portion is 4–5 ounces. Three or more each week = 1 point. (*We eat two portions.*)

11. How many times a week do you eat commercial pastry, cookies, pies, puddings, ice cream, etc.? Less than three times per week = 1 point. (*We eat this less than once each month.*)

12. How many times do you eat nuts each week? (A portion is ¹/₂ ounce.) Once or more a week = 1 point. (*We eat about one portion each week.*)

13. Do you usually eat chicken or turkey rather than red meat? Yes = 1 point. (*We almost always eat chicken and turkey instead of red meat.*)

14. How many times each week do you eat vegetables, pasta, or rice with

a sauce that includes onions and garlic sautéed in olive oil? Two or more = 1 point. (*We eat this about five times each week.*)

Realize that if you score 14 points, it does not mean you are eating an ideal diet. For example, the criterion of eating red meat less frequently than once per day is not good enough in my opinion. The scale was simplified from a scale with several answers to each question. I would eat less meat and fewer sweets than one would need to meet the criterion on this scale. However, the scale is still a good check. You should do it monthly for the first six months. You should also use it for troubleshooting if you start to gain weight. My wife and I each scored 12 out of 14 on this scale. We do not eat enough fruit, and we do not eat enough fish. In each case, we are close to meeting the criterion. We eat two pieces of fruit each day, and eat fish two times each week, on average.

You just may not be able to conform to this scale for individual reasons such as you cannot tolerate olive oil, or are allergic to fish. In these cases, there are variations of the diet that will work for you. Substituting canola oil for olive oil should work fine. You will probably be okay focusing on poultry and not eating fish, but not if you substitute red meat for fish.

If you just use the scale to evaluate your performance, it is not that great. Your weight is a better indicator, although it trails in time. What you eat this week will begin to show in your weight next week. The best use of this is to see where you need to improve. On the questions where your score is zero, you should move toward compliance.

A score of 12 is pretty good. However, it is not okay to score 12 but eat a pint of rich ice cream each day (which would cause you to miss on 6, too much cream, and 11, too much ice cream). The scale is very simplified. If you miss on questions about saturated fat (5 and 6) or on sugar and sweets (7 and 11), it definitely matters how much you miss by.

Even a score of 14 does not absolutely guarantee you will lose weight, but if your score is 5, you are going to be a lot less likely to lose weight. The numbers on the scale are not an exact prescription. They represent a set of limits. For example, the scale indicates less than one portion of red meat per day. This does not mean you should eat 3.5 ounces of red meat daily. We eat much less than that, and we eat more vegetables than the scale requires.

MEASURING YOUR EXERCISE

You should always consult your physician before starting any new exercise program but, the bare minimum to balance your exercise and diet is a thirty-minute walk four days a week. This is pushing it on the low end. It is less than most researchers believe is necessary to enable weight loss, but all of the studies have been done by combining exercise with reduced-calorie diets. I was able to lose weight on my diet plus as little as thirty minutes four times per week, but I recommend a brisk forty-five-minute walk five days per week. This does not have to be done all at one time, and it does not have to be separate from your daily life. Depending on where you live, you could walk to work or the store. As long as the weather is not too hot, you won't need a shower when you get there.

Many people have suggested that the problems of obesity are less in Europe than in the United States because the Europeans walk more. Many of their cities are laid out in a way that makes walking convenient or even necessary. During a recent trip to Europe, my wife and I walked to and in museums, restaurants, and stores. In spite of the fact that we spent time in the United Kingdom and Ireland and had to deviate somewhat from our diet, neither of us gained an ounce on the seventeen-day trip.

The objective of walking is not just to burn calories. You would need to spend a lot of time exercising to burn off enough calories to make much of a difference. Four thirty-minute brisk walks would burn in the range of 600 calories. A pound of fat is equal to about 3,500 excess calories. Thus, even if your food intake did not compensate for the calorie loss, which is likely, it would take six weeks to walk off a pound at that rate.

While there is no definitive evidence, it appears that the critical function of exercise is to work along with a proper diet to help move your set point to a healthier level, and to keep it there. Certainly there is a considerable amount of evidence suggesting that reduced activity levels are related to the obesity epidemic. My own experience is that my exercise level has a close relationship to my weight. But it is necessary to combine the exercise with proper eating. I weigh less now than I did five years ago when I exercised considerably more. But, as I stay with the diet, my weight drops as my exercise increases.

I recommend that you maintain a diary of your exercise, although I admit that this is something that I have not done. A good place to do so is right on your daily weight chart. This has the advantages of being easy and keeps the data all in one place. When you see missing days you will know it is time to exercise. The chart will enable you to see the impact of your exercise on your overall effort to lose weight.

I expect that if the eating program recommended by *The Laguna Beach Diet* is not working for you, that insufficient exercise is very likely to be the problem. You can consult this exercise record if you have problem losing weight, or if you begin to regain weight you previously lost.

TROUBLESHOOTING

If you are not losing weight, there are two possibilities: 1) this process will not work for you, or 2) you are not following the process. To begin the troubleshooting process, use the diet scale above to identify any discrepancies, and consult your exercise log. Make a list of discrepancies, and try to place them in the order of how important you think they are. This may seem unsystematic, but intuitive approaches are often best when you have to make a very complex decision. You lack a method to make a systematic decision anyway. And you are only deciding what to work on first.

Now you may think that your task is complete. You just have to correct the problem. In some cases this may be true. For example, you may not have realized that you needed to consume two tablespoons of olive oil each day, and consumed less to reduce your caloric intake. In such a case, it may be easy to directly correct the problem. But even in this case, there is a *reason* for the discrepancy, and you should make sure that you understand what it is by using the approach described below.

It is usually easier to correct discrepancies when we understand the reason. Often the solution becomes trivially easy when we understand the reason. In business, we call this "root cause analysis." As an example, I worked with a manager in Silicon Valley who managed the final testing of his company's product. Based on the number of staff and testing machines, his production should have been much higher. He assumed his employees were working too slowly, but his efforts to motivate them had been unsuccessful.

To meet his goals, he was going to have to buy expensive machines and add staff, which made no sense to him.

When we looked for the cause of the slow production, we discovered that the production was slow only in the hour before and the hour after shift change. Further investigation determined that each operator would start to close out his shift and fill out forms in the last half hour and the new operator would take another half hour to get everything ready to start the next shift. Finding this root cause made the solution easy. We designed a method so that production was not stopped at shift change and the production goals were easily met without adding machines or staff. Incidentally, this saved the company in excess of 100 thousand dollars, which was considerably more than my consulting fee.

You may find that your diet and exercise regime is just fine when you're at home, but when you travel for business, both go off course. You eat steak or fast food every day and the only exercise you get is walking from your car to the hotel room. Some actions might work to help keep you on course. Learn some yoga or tai chi (a type of slow-motion exercise that concentrates on movement and proper breathing) that can be done in the privacy of your room without disturbing your neighbors and that does not require luggage space for extra shoes and equipment. Instead of steak and potatoes have some fish with vegetables. Chapter 7 on Eating in Restaurants will enable you to find a healthy lunch, even at some fast food chains. The key point is that there was a reason for going off course and positive actions you can take to correct it.

A simple approach to finding root causes is to use a thinking tool called the Five Whys. You begin with the discrepancy and ask, "Why?" You take the answer and again ask, "Why?" For example, my wife and I fall a bit short on eating fish, being closer to twice each week than to the three listed in the scale.

1. Why don't we eat three portions of fish per week?

   Answer: The fish in my local markets is not that good, and it is too far to drive to get the good fish.

2. Why do you not like the fish from the local markets?

   Answer: The less expensive fish often tastes fishy, and the expensive fish sometimes tastes fishy. If I buy the expensive fish and it is not good, I feel cheated.

Here, there are several approaches. I could ask why I am so sensitive to being ripped off, but I think a better question is:

3. Why can't you select fresh fish?

   Answer: I do not know how to. I have read a little, but never had any coaching.

4. What does your reading tell you?

   Answer: That the texture of a fillet should be firm and the smell should not be "fishy."

5. What is wrong with that?

   Answer: I am reluctant to ask to feel or smell the fish.

Touching packaged fish is okay. Touching the fresh fish flesh would be a problem. On the other hand it is difficult to smell the packaged fish, but

QUALITY CONTROL METHODS HAVE WIDE APPLICATION

The Five Whys is a method that derives from the field of quality control. The modern science of quality control really began in Japan in the 1950s when Dr. W. Edwards Deming went to teach the theory and methods of quality control to the industrial leaders of Japan. They learned well, and Japan became the world leader in manufacturing quality through the application of these teachings. Toyota's domination of the auto industry is a testament to the power of these methods. The Deming Prize is awarded annually in Japan for achievements in quality. While these methods were originally focused on manufacturing, they can be applied very successfully to any process, including weight loss.

I expect that most markets would let me smell the fresh, unpackaged fish. In fact, as a result of going through this exercise, I have been asking to smell the fish before I buy it. This is working well. The markets are fine with it, and the fish I have purchased has been consistently excellent.

This is not rocket science, but before going through this exercise, I would not have seen what the problem was. One of the nice things about eating beef was that there were a couple of markets that I could always trust to have good beef. The variability of fish in most markets is much greater because fish is so much more perishable and vulnerable to handling problems.

For many people, cooking fish is a problem. Usually they overcook it, which destroys the texture and the taste. To do it right takes some experience, but using the proper method is also important. For me, pan-roasting is the simplest, cooking one side in an ovenproof skillet with olive oil and perhaps onion and garlic, then turning the fish over and finishing it in the oven. Grilling is also good. Either way, the fish should just reach the stage where it flakes.

Since the other place my wife and I fall short is on fruit, we can look at another example of the Five Whys:

1. Why do you not eat three pieces of fruit each day?

    Answer: That seems like a lot of fruit. There is a lot of fruit I don't like much. Also, we would have to keep a lot of fruit on hand. That is six pieces per day for the two of us.

2. Why are there so few alternatives?

    Answer: When I think about it, there are lots of fruits. I like apples, bananas, mangos, tomatoes, peaches, strawberries, and plums to name a few. (For those of you who believe that tomatoes are vegetables, note that tomatoes are botanically a fruit, since they are a plant ovary, containing seeds. Politically, however, they are a vegetable. In 1893 the U.S. Supreme Court determined that the tomato was a vegetable. This provided protection for domestic tomato growers, since imported fruits were duty free, while there was a tariff on imported vegetables.) In addition to the above fruits, I also like fruit juices, which would be very convenient to store, and which I do not use at all.

There are many lines you could follow here. The first one I chose below looked good:

3. Why do you not use fruit juices?

Answer: I tend to think of them as artificial, with lots of added sugar.

4. Why do you think that, and is it true?

Answer: I guess I think that because many of them do have added sugar. Although there are many juices that do not have added sugar, they are still usually a way of concentrating the calories and omitting the beneficial fiber.

Concluding that fruit juice is not a good alternative, I move to the next question:

5. Why not use some of the other alternatives?

Answer: I really have not put any creative thought into it. Looking at the definition of fruit, as the ripened ovary of a plant which contains seeds, I realize that there are many more items that I eat regularly that are fruits, including peppers, olives, cucumbers, and avocados. I have tended to think of fruits as being sweet to the taste. That is not an essential property of a fruit. The incorporation of these ingredients into salads is an easy way for me to increase my fruit intake.

In the first case, the root cause I came to was that I was using an improper method to select fish. In that case, my initial assumption was that good fish was often not available. In the second case, I had limited my definition of fruit too much. My initial assumption here was that this was just more fruit than I was comfortable eating. Had I worked from the initial assumptions, I would likely not have corrected the discrepancy. My experience in science and business has seen many examples of the same thing, that finding a more fundamental cause enables the solution of previously intractable problems. I strongly recommend that you use this troubleshooting method to deal with the discrepancies in your weight-loss process. It will take some perseverance, but it may be of enormous help to you.

THE BOTTOM LINE

The point of the book that Pat and I wrote, and the point of this chapter, is that proper measurement not only tells you if the process is succeeding, but it also enables you to correct and improve the process. If weight were our only measure, it would not help very much with course correction. But, by tracking your compliance with the diet and your exercise and charting these along with your weight, you will have a good idea of what you need to do if you are not losing weight. Using a problem-solving tool like the "five whys" assists this course correction. I believe that the tools described here are sufficient to enable a successful process. For the reader interested in a more sophisticated approach to these tools, there are many excellent books on the topic. The classic book is *Guide to Quality Control: Industrial Engineering & Technology* (Asian Productivity Organization, 1986) by Kaoru Ishikawa, but there are many more books available on this topic at the bookstore of the American Society for Quality (www.asq.org).

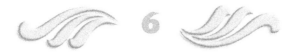

The Mediterranean Diet and Health

6

WHILE A CLEAR PURPOSE of the Laguna Beach Diet is to enable people to lose weight, the ultimate objective is better health. It is worth noting that the healthiest weight may not be cosmetically ideal. You may think you would look better if you were thinner, but if your body mass index (BMI) is around 25, the process I recommend will probably not enable you to lose much weight. (To determine your BMI, see Chapter 2.)

If you want a short, vivid, and entertaining demonstration of the powerful and immediate influence of diet on health, I suggest you watch the movie *Supersize Me.* It depicts the dramatic deterioration in the health of a young man, Morgan Spurlock, who ate only at McDonald's for one month. His body mass index went from 23.9 to 27.0. His cholesterol increased by 50 percent. His liver became so fatty that his physicians were concerned about long-term damage. He also experienced depression and sexual dysfunction.

Remember that this is entertainment, not a scientific experiment. There have been numerous individuals who claim to have lost weight eating at McDonald's. However, they chose salads, not the burgers, fries, and large sodas that represent the bulk of McDonald's sales. Spurlock ate the burgers and fries, which were full of saturated fat, and the large sodas, which contained substantial quantities of high-fructose corn syrup. He did not try to limit calories, and apparently ate even if he was not hungry. It is predictable that this diet would have the effects it did. The only surprise is how quickly the effect developed.

It is also important to note that Spurlock was able to reverse these effects. They were not permanent. While this is not an indictment of McDonald's, it is a strong indictment of a diet of burgers, fries, and sodas.

This chapter will take a more scientific approach than Morgan Spurlock took, and will be less dramatic. More important, it will be different from most writing on nutrition, which typically explains the merits of various foods. If I were writing a book like that, it would be a simple, though tedious, matter to construct an encyclopedia of nutrition. I might tell you that *levo-oxymonium,* found in the stems of rutabagas, enhances the release of insulin in males over sixty-seven years old. (Do not go looking for rutabagas; I made this up.) In fact, some people try to construct a diet using this approach, choosing all sorts of things that some study has found to have a health benefit. My father used to eat dried garlic for its benefit to cardiac health, much to the dismay of anyone in his proximity.

Thus, not only is an item-by-item approach to healthy eating expensive and time-consuming, but it is also fundamentally flawed. A diet is a system and the parts interact. Just because a study showed a beneficial effect of rutabaga stems does not mean that they will work for you. For example, you may eat kiwi fur because it increases the enzymes in your saliva (another made-up story) and it may turn out that kiwi fur inhibits the beneficial effect of rutabaga stems. In a real diet, the interactions are hopelessly complex.

A leading nutritional scientist (quoted from the *European Journal of Epidemiology*) said it this way: "The classical analytical approach has been to assess the exposure to single nutrients or isolated food items, whereas a growing interest exists in studying overall dietary patterns because food items and nutrients could have synergistic or antagonistic effects when they are consumed in combination."

This is not to suggest that most of what nutritionists have to say about individual ingredients is wrong. Much of it is correct and important. But working item-by-item is not an efficient way to construct a diet. Therefore, this chapter is focused on the effects of the Mediterranean Diet on health. That means the whole diet, not the parts. This is a real diet, eaten by real people, over many years. Because it varies from country to country (the food in Crete is different from that in Southern Italy) scientists have

WHEN CONSIDERING ACTION, YOU MUST CONSIDER THE WHOLE SYSTEM

Any complex process, be it a diet, a football play, or a business strategy, should to be viewed as a system. This means that the interactions of the parts need to be taken into account. Failure to do this can leave you vulnerable to unintended consequences that can be very negative. A prominent example of this is the unwanted side effects of drugs. Because the body is an extremely complex system, it is to be expected that a potent drug will have a multitude of effects beyond the intended therapeutic benefit. And because the system is so complex, it is difficult to predict all of these effects in advance. A simple example is antibiotics, intended to kill harmful bacteria. The drugs can also kill the benign bacteria in the intestines and cause digestive problems. Peter Senge's classic *The Fifth Discipline: The Art and Practice of the Learning Organization* (Doubleday, 1990), which applies this theory to organizations, is a good source for more information.

deduced a set of principles that unify the various versions of the diet. These principles are depicted in Chapter 1, and are the basis of my recommendations in *The Laguna Beach Diet.*

An example of an important interaction in foods is the interaction between tomatoes and olive oil. Tomatoes contain lycopene, a powerful antioxidant. The antioxidant effect is significantly increased when the tomatoes are cooked in olive oil. This is, of course, a happy accident for lovers of Italian cooking, rather than the clever design of a nutritionist. The antioxidant capacity of lycopene is thought to be important in the prevention of cardiovascular disease.

The next section presents research showing the effects of the Mediterranean Diet on a number of important health conditions. This is not meant to be an exhaustive compilation, but it serves to show the health benefits of the Laguna Beach Diet.

CARDIOVASCULAR DISEASE

Remember, the diet principles I am recommending originated with research on health, not weight loss. The notion that the Mediterranean Diet is beneficial, derives originally from the Seven Countries Study (discussed in Chapter 2). This study followed 12,763 men for a period of twenty-five years. They were aged forty to fifty-nine at the beginning of the study, which would have made the survivors sixty-five to eighty-four at the end. The study measured deaths from coronary heart disease (CHD), of which there were 5,793 in the study period.

The men came from sixteen areas spread across seven countries. The rates of death (adjusted for age) were dramatically different for the different locations. The death rates in East Finland were five times as high as the death rates in Crete. Southern Italy, and the Japanese groups, also had very low death rates, while the U.S. groups had death rates almost as high as Finland.

A subsequent analysis of the data attributed most of these differences to differences in the consumption of saturated fat, mainly from the consumption of meat and dairy products. The higher the consumption of saturated fat was, the higher the death rate. The authors of this subsequent analysis assert that "the results of the Seven Countries Study show that through a healthy diet and non-smoking, CHD mortality can largely be eliminated from the population before age 70."

While the case above is made in elegant fashion, there are limitations to what can be achieved by this kind of epidemiological study. The problem is that the people in the different cohorts may be different in ways other than diet. These differences may include different genes, different social structures, different activity levels, different access to medical care, ad infinitum. While the researchers can attempt to control such factors statistically, they can never do this completely.

What is required is an experimental study in which all the people are equal. You start with a single group and then randomly assign them to different treatment conditions. If the groups respond differently, you can conclude with some level of statistical certainty that it was the different treatments that led to the different outcomes. Of course it is possible that, by chance, you assigned the healthier people to one group and the sicker people to the other. The statistical computation tells you the probability that luck could have led to the result. A probability value of .001 indicates that the probability that luck caused the effect you observed is 1 in 1,000. The typical criterion for deciding a result is real is a probability value of .05 (5 in 100), or sometimes the more stringent .01 (1 in 100). Most of what I am reporting here is beyond a .001 probability. That means the probability that the health effect resulted from chance rather than the effect of the diet process is less than 1 in 1,000. In this case, you can be very confident of the result.

Fortunately, there are a number of such controlled studies with random assignment of the subjects to the different treatment conditions. One of the most interesting is a study called the Lyon Heart Study conducted in Lyon, France. It is important because of the long follow-up period. Researchers took 605 patients who presented with a nonfatal heart attack and randomized them into two groups. The control group was given instruction on a "prudent Western-type diet similar to the one recommended by the American Heart Association" while the experimental group was given instructions on a typical Mediterranean Diet. The patients were then followed for nearly four years. The rate of deaths from heart attack for the control group was 5.55 per 100 persons per year after twenty-seven months. The rate for a Mediterranean-diet group was 1.24 per 100 persons per year.

If you add major coronary health problems, like heart failure and unstable angina (a type of chest pain resulting from lack of blood flow to the heart muscle that is associated with a high probability of heart attacks), the control group had ninety such incidents over the four years of the study while the Mediterranean-diet group had only twenty-seven. The authors noted that the protective effect of the Mediterranean Diet was powerful and prolonged.

Equally interesting was the ease with which the diet was accepted and followed. The authors noted that many physicians feel that it is easier to prescribe drugs than to change dietary habits. The patients in this study were "closely following the Mediterranean Diet. . . ." They remarked "the adoption of and compliance with new dietary habits is not so difficult, provided that the instruction of the patients (and of their families) and surveillance are properly (professionally) conducted. Of course, the new dietary habits need to be financially and gastronomically acceptable and feasible for patients and their relatives who often have to adapt to a difficult working environment and the stressful urban way of life."

The authors of the study are reinforcing a critical point that I have made about this diet: It can represent a new way of life, and it doesn't have to be difficult to adopt that way of life.

The study includes data on the BMI of the subjects at the end of the study. Both groups were, on average, slightly overweight: The Mediterranean-diet group had an average BMI of 26.3, and the prudent diet group had a 26.9 average. For a person at five feet eight inches tall, this would represent a difference of about 4 pounds, from say 173 to 177. The difference was not significant. One of the things that was surprising is that there was no mention of physical activity. I would not expect a Mediterranean Diet to be very effective in weight loss without an activity component. Nevertheless, neither group average was close to the level of obesity.

Even though the Mediterranean-diet group did not achieve an ideal weight, they appear to have achieved a superior quality of life. Counting all clinical heart incidents (including deaths, major incidents, and minor inci-

SOME PERSPECTIVE ON THE LYON HEART STUDY

Cautious researchers (Kris-Etherton, et al., as reported in *Circulation*) criticized the Lyon Heart Study, based on the fact that it was not entirely clear what diet was eaten by the control group because it was not traced through the study, and there was only limited data on exactly what the Mediterranean-diet group ate. Nevertheless, even the critics noted that "It would be short-sighted to not recognize the enormous public health benefit that this diet would confer with adoption by the population-at-large if the findings are confirmed." I am less cautious at this point, given the mass of evidence supporting the diet. The authors of the Lyon study actually discontinued it before they planned, since they felt it was inappropriate to deny the control group the benefits of a Mediterranean Diet.

dents), the Mediterranean-diet group had ninety-five incidents while the prudent diet group had one hundred eighty. Not only was this nearly twice as many, it was nearly one incident for every person. Of course that does not mean that one hundred eighty people had an incident, as some had more than one. This represents a rather dramatic reduction of heart disease in the Mediterranean-diet group.

METABOLIC SYNDROME

When you measure heart attacks, they are not frequent, even in relatively unhealthy groups. Therefore, the studies often have to use a large number of patients and a long observation period in order to observe clear treatment effects. This is arduous and expensive. Consequently, many studies have measured things that predict heart attacks, such as cholesterol levels and blood pressure. In fact, the National Institutes of Health (NIH) has defined a set of symptoms that, as a group, represent risk factors for heart attack, stroke, kidney failure, and type 2 diabetes. This complex of symptoms is called "metabolic syndrome." The NIH has defined it as having three or more of the following symptoms:

- Waist circumference of more than 40 inches in men and 35 inches in women. (Abdominal obesity has been determined to be a more accurate measure of risk than is BMI, although the two are obviously strongly correlated.)

- Triglycerides level of 150 milligrams per deciliter (mg/dl) or above.

- High-density cholesterol (HDL, the "good" cholesterol) less than 40 mg/dl in men and 50 mg/dl in women.

- Blood pressure of 130/85 mm Hg or above.

- Fasting blood sugar of 100 mg/dl or more.

Other organizations have made adjustments to this definition and have used some different measures, but this is sufficient for our purposes. Now if you have this condition, it may not be cause for panic. In his book *The Last Well Person,* Dr. Nortin Hadler notes that, based on a recent Finnish study, perhaps we should reserve the term metabolic syndrome for "individuals in the top quarter of the population . . . since little risk was established for the remainder." An important point of Hadler's book is that there has been a tendency to bring more and more people into treatment, particularly with pharmaceuticals, by lowering the criteria for what should be treated. His argument is that there is often little or no benefit to treating individuals who just meet the lowered criteria, and that such treatment is expensive and may even carry its own risks.

I agree with Dr. Hadler. However, I think we could also agree that at some level, each of the above symptoms represents a health risk, even if it does not rise to a level justifying treatment with drugs. More than that, I expect that someone with metabolic syndrome has a reduced quality of life. While perhaps we should use medications less frequently to reduce these symptoms, simple dietary changes that reduce the symptoms should be considered beneficial and very worthwhile. In my own case, diet had an impact on several of these variables. I was able to stop taking Lipitor and maintained my total cholesterol at around 200 mg/dl while my HDL has risen from 45 to 57. My waist circumference has dropped from more than 39 inches to under 37 inches. My blood pressure dropped from approximately 135/85 to 120/75 mm Hg, although I continue to use medication. I have more energy and feel better. My triglycerides dropped from 87 to 62 mg/dl, and my blood glucose which is steady at just under 100 has always been within the normal range.

I did not have metabolic syndrome. However, the impact of a Mediterranean Diet on people who actually are diagnosed with the condition is profound. A recent study tested 180 patients with metabolic syndrome

THE PREVALENCE OF METABOLIC SYNDROME

While metabolic syndrome may sound esoteric, this is a rather common condition. It has been estimated that 27 percent of U.S. adults, aged twenty to seventy-four, meet the criteria for this, with the prevalence increasing with age. Over 6 percent of adolescents meet the criteria.

over a two-year period. About half were men and half were women. The average age was about fifty. Half were randomly assigned to a Mediterranean Diet and half to a "prudent diet" with the same proportions of fat, protein, and carbohydrates. Both groups increased their exercise levels to about the same degree.

After two years the Mediterranean-diet group had lost more weight (an average of 9 pounds compared to 2.5 pounds), improved their cholesterol levels more, reduced their waist circumference more, decreased their blood pressure more, and decreased their blood glucose more. The bottom line is that at the end of two years, seventy-three of the ninety patients in the prudent diet group still had metabolic syndrome, while only thirty of the ninety in the Mediterranean-diet group still had metabolic syndrome. This is a huge effect from a relatively simple intervention. Not only did the diet reduce risk, but it also must have made a substantial improvement in the quality of life.

DIABETES

One of the components of metabolic syndrome is a fasting blood glucose level above 100 mg/dl. Depending upon how much above 100 mg/dl it is, it may be a pre-diabetic condition or actual type 2 diabetes. (The American Diabetes Association recommends 126 mg/dL as the level for diagnosis.) The incidence of diabetes has increased dramatically along with the increase in overweight and obesity. It is estimated that in 2005, 9.6 percent of U.S. adults over twenty suffered from diabetes, and 20.9 percent of adults over sixty were diabetic. It is further estimated that 90 to 95 percent of this is type 2 diabetes.

The potential complications of diabetes are quite severe and include a two to fourfold increase in the probability of a heart attack. Other complications include blindness, loss of mental function, kidney disease, and amputation.

Epidemiological studies indicate that a Mediterranean Diet and light exercise are both effective in preventing or delaying the development of this condition. A controlled experiment over a two-year period demonstrated that a Mediterranean Diet reduced insulin resistance compared with a prudent, medically designed diet. Since insulin resistance is an early stage in the development of type 2 diabetes, this provides experimental confirmation that a Mediterranean Diet will decrease the likelihood of developing this awful condition.

CANCER

The World Health Organization (WHO) estimates that 30 percent of worldwide cancer occurrence is related to diet. The evidence shows that a Mediterranean Diet is associated with a low risk of cancer including breast, prostate, and colon cancers. The European Prospective Investigation into Cancer and Nutrition, called the EPIC study, followed more than half a million (520,000) patients in nine European countries over ten years. In one analysis, they scored patients on adherence to a Mediterranean Diet on a 9-point scale similar to the one presented in Chapter 5. They found that for every 2-point increase in compliance with a Mediterranean Diet, there was a 24 percent reduction in deaths from cancer.

Analysis of the EPIC data showed that increased consumption of dietary fiber (found in whole gains and fresh fruits and vegetables), and consumption of fish led to a reduction of colorectal cancer. Increased consumption of red meat and processed meat (like bacon, lunch meat, and smoked meats) was related to an increased incidence of colorectal cancer. Increased consumption of fruit was associated with a decreased incidence of lung cancer. The study also showed that being overweight was related to an increased incidence of cancer deaths.

While the EPIC study is a prospective study, meaning that patients were followed over a period of time after the study began, it is not a controlled experimental study with random assignment to conditions. However, there is one relevant experimental study, the Lyon Heart Study that I discussed in the context of cardiovascular disease. This involved the same 605 patients, randomized into a Mediterranean-diet group or a prudent diet group. During the four-year follow-up, seventeen of the prudent diet group and seven of the Mediterranean-diet group were diagnosed with cancer. When cancers diagnosed in the first two years of follow-up were omitted, based on the idea that the influence of the new diets would take some time to emerge, the numbers were twelve cancers for the prudent diet group and only two for the Mediterranean-diet group. While the results were statistically significant, the authors felt that more research with more patients and/or longer follow-up periods was needed to confirm the cancer-protective effect of a Mediterranean Diet. Since numerous researchers in the field have also noted the need for additional research, it is very likely that this research is currently in progress. In the meantime, given the powerful epidemiological evidence, confirmed by the only controlled experiment, it is reasonable to assume that a Mediterranean Diet does have a cancer-protective effect.

ALZHEIMER'S DISEASE

In my age group the greatest health worry is not obesity, heart disease, diabetes, or even cancer. Most conversations with my peers about aging include a statement about the fear of Alzheimer's disease. While the causes are unknown, diet appears to have an important effect. A study recently published in *Archives of Neurology* suggests that adherence to a Mediterranean Diet profoundly reduces the risk of Alzheimer's disease. While the study was not a controlled experiment, the results are convincing. The study followed a population of 1,790 non-demented people and 194 patients with Alzheimer's disease, matched to each other on a number of variables. Researchers measured adherence to a Mediterranean Diet on a 9-point scale. This is similar to the scale presented in Chapter 5. Patients with scores of 7 and above were 60 percent less likely to have Alzheimer's disease than patients with scores of 3 and below. Each point on the 9-point scale reduced the risk of Alzheimer's disease by 19 to 24 percent. If this is not enough to motivate you to move in the direction of a Mediterranean-style diet, it would certainly be enough for me. Fortunately, I moved there more than three years ago.

PERIODONTAL DISEASE

One of the most surprising experiences I had since beginning to eat according to the principles of a Mediterranean Diet came when I had a routine periodontal examination. For at least five years I had a persistent level of problems, as diagnosed by the hygienist at each visit. The diagnosis involved inserting a probe between the tooth and the gum and measuring the depth from the gum margin to the bone. This, by the way, is not my favorite way to spend time. I had several areas where the depth was consistently too great. Year after year the problems did not get better and did not get worse. The problem was not bad enough to require treatment, but needed to be watched carefully in case it progressed. Suddenly there was a marked improvement. I was inclined to attribute this to my new diet, but obviously had no scientific basis to do so.

In consulting the scientific literature, I could find no studies on the effect of a Mediterranean Diet on periodontal health. There was, however, massive literature on the relationship between cardiovascular disease and periodontal disease. The two conditions are highly correlated. The assumption of most writers was that periodontal disease was a causative factor in cardiovascular disease. However, I did find one epidemiological study that suggested that both conditions were influenced by a more fundamental set of factors: body mass index, physical exercise, and diet. Individuals who met the authors' criteria for these actions for normal BMI, sufficient exercise, and healthy eating were 16 percent less likely to have periodontal disease. Of course, it is well established that these same activities also prevent cardiovascular disease. Since the Mediterranean Diet qualifies as a form of healthy eating, the study provides some support for my hypothesis that my own condition improved as a result of my change in diet.

Let me admit that this analysis is a bit labored. What is needed is an experimental study of the impact of the Mediterranean Diet on periodontal disease. Although periodontal disease seems a lot less important than heart disease and cancer, I mention it for two reasons: 1) since periodontal disease is the main cause of tooth loss in adults, it is important, and 2) this demonstrates how wide the range is of health effects that may accrue to someone who adopts this diet.

THE BOTTOM LINE

A trite quotation is "you are what you eat." Certainly it is not surprising that what you eat has a huge impact on your health. What is surprising to me is the powerful health-enhancing effect of the Mediterranean Diet, even when it is compared to a prudent Western-style diet that is very similar in its caloric content and its relative proportions of fat, protein, and carbohydrate. A Mediterranean-style diet is superior in protecting against cardiovascular disease, diabetes, kidney disease, stroke, several forms of cancer, Alzheimer's disease, and perhaps even periodontal disease. Not only is it protective, but it can also reverse some of the symptoms of cardiovascular disease in people who have already had heart attacks or who have been diagnosed with metabolic syndrome. This is a very simple intervention compared to the pharmaceutical and surgical interventions often employed to deal these conditions.

Eating in Restaurants

 EATING IN RESTAURANTS IS A FACT of life for most people. Fortunately for me, I have the time and inclination to cook, but my wife and I still find ourselves in a restaurant two to three times each week. Of course, when we travel, we eat all our meals in restaurants. Our last vacation was seventeen days and included airline food along with restaurants in the United Kingdom, Ireland, and southern Spain. While southern Spain is a Mediterranean region, the United Kingdom and Ireland might be classified as "anti-Mediterranean." Still, with the globalization of cuisine, and with some thought to what we ordered, we were able to negotiate the entire trip with no weight gain, and with considerable food enjoyment at the same time. Our diet was inferior to what we eat at home, but this Mediterranean-diet process is sufficiently robust to deal with the divergence.

SELECTING THE RIGHT KIND OF RESTAURANT

The first challenge is choosing where to eat. When I select a restaurant, it has to meet three requirements: 1) the menu has to offer healthy choices; 2) the food has to be good; and 3) the value for the money has to be good, meaning that if the restaurant is expensive, the food has to be really good.

Finding healthy choices is easier if you choose the right kind of restaurant. Restaurants likely to have more menu choices that are healthy:

• Italian

- Asian

- Seafood

- Middle Eastern

- Mom and pop restaurants that cook from fresh ingredients

Restaurants that are likely to have fewer healthy choices:

- Fast food

- Most large chains

- Steakhouses

- Barbecue

- Mexican

Choosing a restaurant from the first list does not guarantee a healthy meal, and you can probably find something relatively healthy on the restaurants on the second list. I will explain more later when I get into details about menu items.

Choosing a restaurant that has good food and value is tricky. It has taken years of travel and living in many places for me to develop this skill. Here is an example of an outing that we took the weekend before I wrote this. We traveled, with another couple, to an exhibition opening at the art museum in Oceanside, California, about twenty miles north of our home. Oceanside is a military town, dominated by the Camp Pendleton Marine base. It is principally a working-class town, although the beach area is becoming very upscale.

While walking from the parking lot to the museum I noticed a sign on a storefront Vietnamese restaurant, the Wok Inn. The sign welcomed guests to celebrate the twentieth anniversary of the restaurant. Two things struck me about this. First, the restaurant had survived twenty years, so it must be okay. Second, the proprietors were obviously proud of their restaurant. One of the things I look for is a sense of pride in the proprietors, which is usually revealed in the decorations and cleanliness.

I checked the menu and looked in the door. The menu was interesting, combining Vietnamese, Thai, and Chinese dishes. This is pretty common in Vietnamese restaurants here. The place was bright, cheery, and clean, though a bit on the eclectic side, which is also common in Vietnamese restaurants. Actually, what is eclectic to me is probably not at all eclectic to a Vietnamese person. At any rate, after we viewed the art at the museum, we took our friends back to the restaurant and had a lovely meal. We were given free champagne to celebrate the anniversary, along with some free appetizers. The champagne was okay. This was not gourmet food mind you, but our friends, who have traveled extensively, thought it was the best Pad Thai (a Thai-style noodle dish) they had ever had. I could not go that far, but everything was quite good. The bill, before the tip, was about twenty dollars per couple. Of course, if the food were not good, it would be a bad deal even at half the price, but this was a tremendous bargain. Since we go to the Oceanside museum on a regular basis, we will definitely be returning to that restaurant.

In choosing a restaurant, there are several things to look for. The first impression is the outside. It does not have to be attractive, but it should not be run down. Walking in the front door, you should see that it is clean and orderly, and here your intuition goes to work. Predicting food quality from the way a restaurant looks and smells is a very complex problem. The process requires more than simple logic. You really cannot do it with a checklist, so trusting your intuition is usually best.

If I am satisfied with my impression, I look at the menu. First, is it clean or are there food and beverage stains. Second, does it have anything interesting or somewhat unique. In general, I prefer a menu with unique or rarely offered menu items. One, this indicates that the restaurant is preparing food from fresh ingredients rather than purchasing pre-prepared meals and just heating them. Two, it demonstrates that someone has done a bit of thinking about what is being served. In addition to these evaluations, I look to see if there is anything I might like. If I see a dozen beef dishes and one fish and one chicken breast, I suspect that the chef's heart is not really in these latter dishes.

Way up on the list of impressions is the feeling I get about the owner's sense of pride as reflected in the things I have talked about. The reason that pride is important is that it is very likely to be reflected in the quality of the food. One of my most important teachers, Dr. W. Edwards Deming, explained that pride of workmanship is the strongest motivation for doing high quality work. The restaurant that takes pride in its work will have the best food. Many chains, especially the fast food chains, have tried to replace pride of workmanship with systems similar to those used in manufacturing. This is essentially the mass production of food. They have succeeded in producing a uniform product, but not in replacing the food you can get from a cook who has pride of workmanship.

This brings to mind a story. There is a small restaurant in New Haven, Connecticut called Louis' Lunch. The place was established in 1895 and has been in downtown New Haven ever since. It serves hamburgers, steak sandwiches, hot dogs and, on Fridays, tuna salad. I was taken there by friends when I was in college in New Haven in the 1960s. It was a set up. My friends told me nothing about the place, except that it was good. I ordered a hamburger and it was delivered on toasted white bread with an onion. Knowing that I was new, the regulars stopped talking and turned to watch. And I fell right into the trap. I asked for ketchup. This was an insult and the proprietor told me in no uncertain terms that his hamburgers were good the way he served them and that no one would ever bring ketchup into his establishment. He was right on both counts.

I have never seen a clearer case of pride of workmanship than Louis' Lunch. That is why a tiny restaurant has survived for more than 100 years. In the 1970s the city wanted to tear it down for redevelopment. Demonstrations by angry customers ensued. Eventually the historic building was moved to a new location in the downtown area. You can find more details at www.louislunch.com. Although I might be able to make a checklist for evaluating the pride of workmanship that a restaurant represents, I think your intuition will prove to be the best guide.

SELECTING HEALTHY OFFERINGS

When all the tests are passed and I sit down at a table with the menu, I look for menu items that have the proper ingredients, and that are prepared in a healthy way. The following are some of the things to think about:

- Whenever possible, order meals prepared from fresh ingredients. Take advantage of the fresh fruits and vegetables. (Remember, tomatoes and avocados are fruits.)

- Avoid red meat.

- Opt for fish, preferably grilled, but only if the restaurant does a good job with fish. Avoid cream sauces and butter melted on top.

- Opt for chicken. Most restaurants these days have a roasted chicken on the menu. (I recently read about a trendy Los Angeles restaurant that served a rotisserie chicken with an a-la-carte price north of 40 dollars.) Watch out for chickens and chicken breasts treated with sodium (a flavor enhancer and preservative). Ask the restaurant where the chicken comes from. Is it fresh from a butcher or provisioner or prepared and packaged.

- Avoid fried and deep-fried foods. Fried potatoes are okay occasionally, but only if cooked in vegetable oil. Fries cooked in partially hydrogenated oil contain trans fat. These are unhealthy and should not be eaten. Restaurants cite the use of partially hydrogenated oil as a cost savings. Partially hydrogenated oils are more stable, and can be used longer. Most chains, including McDonald's and Burger King, currently produce fries that contain significant levels of trans fat. Baked potato is a better choice, but ask for olive oil rather than butter or sour cream.

- Avoid overcooked, heavily charred, or broiled foods.

- Weed out cheese-laden dishes and sauces made with cream and/or butter.

- Choose minimally prepared vegetables, such as steamed or sautéed, but watch out for the butter.

- Limit amount of oil-based salad dressing you use. Green salads are wonderful, but most of the dressings are not. These oils are almost always refined. The best idea is to ask for vinegar and oil. Most restaurants will give you the cruets and let you dress the salad yourself. Potato and pasta salads are usually made with an abundance of mayonnaise, and generally should be avoided.

- If you do eat cake, cookies, or other confections, eat small portions, and do this infrequently. Avoid ice cream and whipped cream. If you decrease your intake of heavily sweetened foods, fresh fruits will begin to taste much sweeter.

The above recommendations will probably be enough to avoid pre-prepared dishes. Because most of what goes on in restaurants is largely behind the scenes, you should feel free to ask questions.

In my experience, however, there is huge variability and the accuracy of the answers, especially when you are asking the waiter. Many restaurants, especially chains, use pre-prepared entrées. These could be meat, poultry, or even seafood and may include a sauce. These are almost always very high is sodium and may contain trans fat. I contacted the chains Applebee's and Olive Garden and they could not or would not supply nutrition information about their menus. The Applebee's website did have information on their Weight Watchers items and the Olive Garden website had information on their "Garden Fare" selections (menu items that purport to meet the criteria for healthy fare). In neither case did the information include sodium content or saturated fat.

To their credit, another chain, Denny's did provide comprehensive information on their website. I recently ate a grilled chicken sandwich there. It turned out to have a relatively low saturated fat content, but, consistent with what I said above, it had a very high-sodium content, 1,494 milligrams (mg). (A teaspoon of salt is approximately 2,500 mg, and represents the upper limit of what you should eat in a day.) Since the sodium content of the chicken breast itself would be less than 150 mg, it is safe to assume that the processing added nearly half a teaspoon of salt. It is clear that other chains add lots of salt to their chicken breasts. The data from Burger King and McDonald's demonstrates this clearly, even in the grilled chicken they put on their "healthy" salads. While none of the descriptions of the Mediterranean Diet that I have seen specify sodium intake, the diet is based on fresh foods, not processed foods. It is unlikely that these levels of sodium would ever be reached in the preparation of fresh foods.

Italian Restaurants

There is more to choose than avoid. After all, Italy is on the Mediterranean.

- Pasta. Avoid cream sauces and pasta baked with a lot of cheese, unless a lot of that cheese is ricotta. You can eat sauces with a little meat.

- Risotto is probably not a good idea, as it is usually cooked with butter and cream.

- Polenta is okay, but watch out for the butter.

- Choose the chicken and seafood dishes over the beef, lamb, and pork.

Middle Eastern Restaurants

Middle Eastern cuisines tend to be more vegetable based; make liberal use of olive oil, spices, and herbs; use little dairy; and usually include chicken so that you can avoid red meat. (Lamb is like beef, in my opinion.) The vegetarian plates with falafel and hummus are often very good.

- Roasted chicken is always appropriate.

- There are many stews with ingredients like eggplant, lentils, pomegranate, and walnuts to name a few.

- Brown rice is usually not available, but the white rice is okay as long as you are getting fiber elsewhere.

Seafood Restaurants

The current fish story is getting pretty complex. There are concerns about mercury, which is particularly dangerous for women of childbearing age. Fish high in mercury include shark, tuna (canned and fresh), and Chilean sea bass. Some fish contain more essential omega-3 fats than others. These are the fatty fishes like salmon and halibut. As this tends to be too complex to me, I look for what is fresh and a decent value. Since I am eating fish two or three times each week, and my wife and I are not planning any more children, I don't worry about the mercury. Since I like fatty fish, I think I am getting enough omega-3s.

- Grilled fish or fish sandwiches are okay.

- Avoid deep-fried fish and chips, especially because they are likely to be fried in partially hydrogenated oil.

- Pan-roasted fish with a sauce is fine, but avoid sauces based on cream and/or butter.

Mexican Restaurants

Mexican food served in the United States and in the border areas of Mexico frequently has lots of saturated fat. While chicken is always available, beef and pork are more prominent. Refried beans and flour tortillas are traditionally made with lard. The results of all this appears to be reflected in the high incidence of obesity in the young women I see when visiting Ensenada. In fact, however, you can eat healthy meals in most Mexican restaurants by making the right choices.

- Corn tortillas are fine. They are made with corn, water, and a bit of lime. There is no fat. Flour tortillas are not so good, as they are made with white flour and typically contain saturated fat. Mission is a widely sold brand of tortillas here in Southern California. A 12-inch flour tortilla from them contains 2.5 g of saturated fat, which is tolerable. Surprisingly, it also contains 670 mg of sodium, which is more than 25 percent of the recommended daily amount. Compare this with two of their 6-inch corn tortillas, which is close to the same amount of food. The two corn tortillas contain no saturated fat and only 20 mg of sodium (10 mg each).

- Chicken is preferred to beef.

- The rice is usually okay, so long as it is not covered with butter. Brown rice is usually not available.

- Refried beans are often cooked in lard. If so, avoid them. More and more restaurants are using canola oil, and these are fine.

- Sauces like molé (pronounced mol-eh) are fine if prepared with vegetable oil and should be avoided if prepared using lard or butter. Chicken with molé sauce is one of my favorites. In case you are not familiar with molé, it is a blend of chocolate and smoky chillies. Sounds bad, tastes great.

OBESITY APPEARS TO AFFLICT MEXICAN-AMERICAN WOMEN MORE THAN MEXICAN-AMERICAN MEN

Mexican-American women have a much higher rate of obesity than their non-Hispanic white counterparts. The rate for Mexican-American women over twenty is 39.8 percent, rising to 47.9 percent for Mexican-American women in the forty to fifty-nine age group. For non-Hispanic white women, the rates are 30.5 percent and 35.9 percent, respectively. Of course, this could be a result of genes, economic status, activity, and/or diet. Interestingly, Mexican-American men have very slightly lower rates of obesity than non-Hispanic whites. The fact that relatively affluent Mexican women have an obesity rate of 43.1 percent suggests that economics is at least not the sole factor.

- Fish tacos, very popular in southern California and Baja, are excellent. These are usually made with corn tortillas, shredded cabbage, and salsa. Avoid mayonnaise. Chicken tacos are okay but avoid beef tacos.

- Burritos are not as good as tacos because they are made with flour tortillas. Burritos with chicken, beans, rice, and salsa filling are a compromise, but contain much more saturated fat than tacos.

Asian Restaurants

First, try to find an Asian restaurant that does not use the flavor enhancer MSG (monosodium glutamate). In my experience, Japanese, Vietnamese, and Thai restaurants generally have more healthy choices than Chinese restaurants. In many Chinese dishes the meat is deep-fried. Ask what kind of oil they cook in. Canola oil is lighter tasting than olive oil and is best for Asian food. Olive oil might be healthier, but it begins to smoke at the high heat levels used in a wok. Still, stick with the right choices and you can get a healthy meal in most Asian restaurants.

- Favor chicken, duck, and seafood. Make sure that they cook in vegetable oil that is not partially hydrogenated. Canola oil (lighter tasting than olive oil) is best for Asian food.

- Brown rice is preferable to white rice. More and more Asian restaurants in Southern California are offering it.

- Typically, sushi is a good choice, since it has very little fat. However, the California roll, a kind of sushi made with crab, avocado, cucumber that has been influential in inspiring sushi's popularity in America, usually contains a nice dose of cream cheese, and therefore is an exception.

- Seafood and vegetable dishes will have the lowest levels of saturated fat. They tend to use dark meat in the chicken dishes, however, which has more saturated fat than light meat. Also, they frequently include the skin, dramatically raising the saturated fat content for both dark and light meat.

Fast Food

Fast food is a fact of modern life. Understanding it is important, as it is difficult to avoid completely. I have always liked McDonald's burgers, so my resistance to fast food in general is based on nutritional information, not flavor and ambiance.

Fast-food restaurants are essentially small, mass-production facilities. They design a food product, which based on extensive testing, appeals to customers. Then they develop an assembly line process to manufacture it in their restaurants. They purchase uniform raw materials, such as beef, poultry, and potatoes. They, or their vendors, process them into items like hamburger patties, chicken nuggets, and uncooked French fries. The local restaurant assembles these parts into meals, cooking them when necessary. The fact that they tend to call their outlets "stores" rather than "restaurants," emphasizes that only a limited amount of preparation is done on the premises. The intent is to create a product that is not only attractive, but also uniform from store to store. Their huge sales suggest success at the former. My experience indicates that the uniformity is remarkable. I have eaten Big Macs in Hong Kong, and Tokyo, and found them hard to distinguish from the American counterpart.

One characteristic of fast food that is nearly universal is that it contains huge amounts of sodium. This makes their chicken juicy, flavorful, resistant to spoilage, and also much less healthy than it might be. As I mentioned before, the Mediterranean Diet requires that you eat food that is "minimally processed." Most, though not all, fast food is maximally processed. Processing often adds sodium and removes fiber. Trans fat is often added. Many of the chains use partially hydrogenated oil to cook their fries and chicken, although pressure from consumers and health authorities may change this. While fast food may be tasty, convenient, and economical, much of it is not healthy.

When I am cooking, I generally do not worry about nutritional content. I simply use the proper ingredients and trust the result. With fast food, many of the steps in preparation are not obvious, and in some cases they are likely to be trade secrets. Therefore, an examination of nutritional data becomes important.

To their great credit, all of the fast food outlets I have checked supply extensive data about their menus on their websites. Table 7.1 on pages 110–111 presents a sampling of this data from four outlets: McDonald's, Burger King, Subway, and El Pollo Loco. The latter is a Mexican chain currently numbering 340 stores in the United States, specializing in flame-broiled chicken, served with tortillas, rice, and beans. The areas shaded in light gray are areas for caution and suggest the items should be avoided. Areas shaded in dark gray are positive and represent the better choices.

The universal feature for all four chains is very high sodium content. Even though El Pollo Loco cooks whole legs and breasts, they are apparently treated in some way to raise the sodium content. The objective would be to enhance the flavor and extend the shelf life of the product. The El Pollo Loco meal of chicken breast, pinto beans, and corn tortillas is pretty good, except for the sodium content, with only 2 grams of saturated fat. There are three other Mexican chains with roots in Southern California: Rubio's, La Salsa, and Baja Fresh. All offer a bit more opportunity for a healthy meal if you choose correctly. Baja Fresh has the tacos with the lowest saturated fat. Focus on the chicken and fish tacos, and skip the burritos and enchiladas. I have yet to find any chain without high sodium.

The Whopper and Big Mac are both whoppers for saturated fat, with 11 and 10 grams of saturated fat respectively. Add the fries and you get a small dose of trans fat as well. Throw in a large cola and you get 86 grams of sugar, which is almost one-fifth of a pound. The Asian salads with chicken combined with the low-fat dressing are a better choice but still have 5 grams of saturated fat and more than 1,500 mg of sodium. Also, I find these salads far less filling than what I am looking for.

TABLE 7.1 • FAST FOOD NUTRITIONAL DATA

RESTAURANT	DISH/FOOD	CALORIES	FAT (g)	% OF CALORIES FROM FAT
El Pollo Loco	chicken breast with skin	187	7	34%
	corn tortilla	210	3	13%
	flour tortilla	330	12	33%
	black beans	308	16	47%
	pinto beans	154	4	23%
	Spanish rice	151	1	6%
	meal of chicken breast, 3 corn tortillas, rice and pinto beans	1,122	21	17%
McDonald's	Premium grilled classic chicken sandwich	420	9	19%
	Big Mac	860	30	31%
	Asian salad with grilled chicken	290	10	31%
	Newman's own low-fat sesame ginger dressing	90	2.5	25%
	meal of Asian salad and low-fat sesame ginger dressing	380	12.5	30%
	medium french fries	390	20	47%
Burger King	Whopper	670	39	52%
	med fries, salted	360	20	50%
	Tendergrill chicken sandwich, no mayo	450	10	20%
	Tendergrill chicken salad	240	9	34%
	Ken's light Italian dressing	120	11	83%
	meal of salad and dressing	360	20	50%
Subway	6" spicy Italian sandwich	227	25	48%
	6" turkey breast sandwich	280	4.5	40%
	6" tuna sandwich	530	31	53%

SATURATED FAT (g)	% OF FAT THAT IS SATURATED	TRANS FAT	CARBS	PROTEIN	SODIUM (mg)	FIBER
2	29%	0	0	30	540	0
0	0%		42	3	105	3
3	25%		48	9	630	3
6	38%		35	7	731	5
0	0%		24	7	674	9
0	0%		33	3	421	1
2	10%		183	49	1,950	19
2	22%	0	52	32	1,240	3
10	33%	1.5	47	25	1,010	14
5	50%	0	23	31	890	6
0	0%	0	14	1	680	0
5	40%	0	37	32	1,570	6
4	20%	5	47	4	220	5
11	28%	1.5	51	28	1,020	3
4.5	23%	4.5	41	4	590	4
2	20%	0	53	37	1,210	4
3.5	39%	0	8	33	720	4
1.5	14%	0	5	0	440	0
5	25%	0	13	33	1,160	4
9	36%	0	45	21	1,660	4
1.5	33%	0	46	18	1,000	4
7	23%	1	44	22	1,010	4

Subway, which probably has a franchise within minutes of most residents of the United States, advertises a line of sandwiches with less than 6 grams of fat. These have very low saturated fat content. The only problem is the universal fast food bogeyman of very high sodium. Surprisingly, their tuna sandwich is not among the healthy choices. It has 31 grams of fat, 7 grams of saturated fat, and even 0.5 grams of trans fat. They must use some potent mayonnaise!

If you must choose fast food, Subway and El Pollo Loco are better choices than the traditional burgers. If you eat at a burger place, look for grilled chicken or grilled fish sandwiches and use mustard instead of mayonnaise. You will probably get a lot of sodium but will likely be okay on saturated fat and trans fat. The salads are statistically okay, but would leave me very hungry.

Pizza

Pizza represents a category of food that is similar to fast food. I would call it convenience food. I love pizza. When I was in college, I would walk across New Haven with my roommates almost every weekday night after studying (or playing bridge) to Sally's Apizza on Wooster Street. It is still the

TABLE 7.2 • PIZZA NUTRITIONAL DATA

RESTAURANT	SERVING SIZE	CALORIES	FAT (g)	% OF CALORIES FROM FAT
Papa John	slice 14" cheese, orig crust, 132 g	300	11	33%
	slice 14" cheese, thin crust, 91 g	240	13	50%
	slice 14" orig crust, pepperoni, 128 g	310	13	39%
Pizza Hut	slice 14" cheese, original crust, 100 g	271	11	36%
UNO	deep dish cheese & tomato, 551 g	1,710	104	55%
Pizza Hut	5 slices to equal amount of pizza in UNO	1,355	55	55%

best pizza I have ever had. Friends in the area have told me that patrons now wait hours for a seat. In my day, a 9-inch cheese pizza was 80 cents. Fortunately for my nutritional condition, Sally's is now 2,500 miles away.

I admit to occasionally eating pizza, but the typical American pizza is not an ideal food for our diet. Table 7.2 below lists nutritional information on pizza from three chains. I do not particularly like their pizza, and do not eat it, but I do not expect the nutritional information is much different for the pizza I like.

The largest source of variation is what each chain considers a "serving" in their nutritional tables. Pizza Hut and Papa John list one slice of a 14-inch pizza, weighing about 100 grams, while UNO lists an individual pizza at 551 grams. (A pound is 454 grams.) I think reality is in between. I am not sure that I, a serious pizza eater, can do five slices of a 14-inch pizza, and I do not like deep dish anyway. If you compare the UNO pizza to five slices of the Pizza Hut, you have two very fatty meals, although the UNO pizza has a lot more. The bottom line is that if you eat several slices, or an individual deep-dish pizza, you are getting a lot of saturated fat, and the usual very large dose of sodium. Adding meat to the pizza does not make a lot of difference, since there is plenty of saturated fat in the cheese. Although

SATURATED FAT (g)	% OF FAT THAT IS SATURATED	TRANS FAT (g)	CARBS (g)	PROTEIN	SODIUM (mg)	FIBER (g)
3.5	32%	0	30	13	750	2
3.5	27%	0	22	10	500	1
4	31%	0	38	13	800	2
4	36%		32	12	632	1
38	37%		119	64	2,260	7
20	36%	0	160	60	3,160	5

pizza is an Italian dish, this kind of pizza is hardly a typical Mediterranean food. My limited experience with pizza in Italy is that the pie is smaller, has a thicker crust than American thin-crust pizza, uses fresh tomatoes and other ingredients, and has much less cheese.

I do still eat pizza occasionally, about once each month. The veggie pizzas tend to have a bit less cheese. Stay away from the deep-dish variety with a thick layer of cheese.

Fine Dining

Fine restaurants have some advantages and disadvantages for the customer attempting to conform to the principles of the Laguna Beach Diet. The largest advantage is that they almost always prepare dishes from fresh ingredients. The largest disadvantage is that they frequently use significant quantities of butter and cream. However, I have yet to find a fine restaurant that does not offer some good choices. Even if you are forced into Ruth's Chris Steakhouse, an upscale chain of steakhouses across the United States, you can order seafood or chicken.

The best restaurant in my town, and one of the best in all of San Diego County, is Pacifica Del Mar. I spoke with the chef de cuisine, Brad Luckenbill, about their menu and specifically about how several of the dishes were prepared.

For example, on the Starters menu, the Dungeness crab cakes looked good, but I was concerned about the fat content. Based on the recipe I estimate that a serving contains approximately 0.2 ounces of cream resulting in about 6 grams of saturated fat. Add the butter in the sauce and this is too high for me. This is the only starter I would reject on a menu that includes pepper-seared ahi (tuna), house-smoked salmon, steamed eastern mussels, tempura prawns, and several others.

On the soups and salads menu, everything is okay. The one question I had was the corn-leek bisque that I expected to contain cream. In fact, it contains some cream cheese, but ends up with approximately 3 grams of saturated fat in a one cup serving, which I find acceptable. Other items on this menu include a baby spinach and arugula salad, hearts of romaine, Japanese clam chowder, and organic mixed greens. The clam chowder contains lots of butter and is not a good choice.

Below is the Entrée section of the Pacifica Del Mar menu, taken from their website. My comments below each item are in italics. The item descriptions are very helpful in making a choice.

Entrées

- **Broiled Maine Lobster**
  Basted with Herb-Garlic Butter, Lobster-Rice Pilaf, Spinach
  (Watch out for the herb-garlic butter.)

- **Filet Mignon**
  Broccolini, Potato-White Cheddar Gratin, Zinfandel Sauce
  (Pass on this because of the cheese and butter in the sauce.)

- **Grilled House Cured Ribeye**
  Portobello Mushrooms, Broccolini, Natural Jus (4.5 grams net carbs for low-carb customers)
  (Again, pass on this because of the generous portion of red meat.)

- **Grilled Opah**
  Orange-Cumin-Honey Glaze, Shiitake, Spring Squash, Smashed Red Potatoes
  (This is an excellent choice with the fish, in spite of a little fat in the glaze.)

- **Herb-Encrusted Whitefish**
  Spinach Gnocchi, Wild Mushrooms, Beurre Blanc, Chile Oil
  (The beurre blanc is loaded with butter, but the rest is okay. You could ask them to go light on the buerre blanc.)

- **House-Cured Ribeye**
  Wild Mushrooms, Haricot Verts, Truffle Cheese-Potato Croquette, and Sherry-Shallot Jus
  (Pass on this dish because of the beef.)

- **Mustard Catfish**
  Chile Marinade, Yukon Potato-Corn Succotash, Green Onion Aioli
  (This is an excellent choice of fish with very little fat anywhere. Very tasty too.)

- **Pacifica's Barbecued Sugar-Spiced Salmon**
  Chinese Beans, Garlic Mashed Potatoes, Mustard Sauce
  (The mashed potatoes and the sugar glaze on the salmon make this less than ideal.)

- **Pan-Roasted Free-Range Chicken Breast**
  Roast Garlic-Noodle Galette, Spicy Roast Tomato Sauce, Balsamic Syrup
  (This is an excellent choice with chicken and relatively low-fat sides.)

- **Pan-Roasted Northern Halibut**
  Tat Soi, Shimeji Mushrooms, Barley, and Szechuan Peppercorn Broth
  (This is an excellent choice with very little saturated fat.)

- **Pan-Seared Atlantic Sea Scallops**
  Cherry Tomatoes, Melted Leeks, Truffled Polenta, and Arugula
  (This is an excellent choice with very little saturated fat.)

- **Pan-Roasted Seabass**
  Soy Glaze, Sticky Rice, Bok Choy, Green Curry-Coconut Sauce
  (This is an excellent choice with a little butter but still low in saturated fat.)

- **Pepper and Coriander Seared Ahi**
  Buttered Carrots, Shiitake-Spinach Strudel, Citrus Ponzu
  (Probably okay, better without the butter on the carrots.)

- **Salt and Pepper Prawns**
  Udon Noodles, Black Bean-Garlic Sauce, Choy Sum, Green Onions
  (This is an excellent choice with very little saturated fat.)

All of their food is prepared from fresh ingredients and the chicken is free-range organic chicken. The cooking oil is canola oil or a combination of 80 percent canola and 20 percent olive oil. The food is even healthier than I expected. In your own dining choices, you will likely have to ask a few questions about ingredients and preparation of dishes that you may want to choose.

Mom and Pop Restaurants

One of the most difficult places to find healthy food is in small mid-western towns. A few years ago I traveled regularly to a town of about 5,000 inhabitants in Iowa. This town, like many others, was dominated by fast food and chains. Beef was king. The best choices turned out to be mom and pop restaurants that processed food from fresh ingredients. Although the chains have driven many of these establishments out of business, the best appear to have survived. Although the bulk of choices are still not ideal, it is at least possible to really know what you are getting. There are usually chicken and fish entrées with fresh vegetables and potatoes.

THE BOTTOM LINE

Although you surrender a lot of control when eating in restaurants, it is not that difficult to make healthy choices. Whenever you are in doubt, ask how the dish is prepared. If you are in a chain or a fast food outlet, they may not know, but they will probably have a nutritional chart that you can consult. Choosing a restaurant that has really good food is more difficult. Here, in the absence of definitive information, trusting your intuition is probably the best approach.

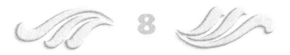

Some Thoughts
on Cooking

I ENJOY COOKING. MY ABILITY TO COOK, and to make a variety of dishes that fit the scheme of the Laguna Beach Diet has been helpful in the process of losing weight and at the same time converting my eating habits. While you can adopt this diet without cooking at all, the ability and inclination to cook is an advantage.

A fundamental element of today's cooking is the recipe. This is a formula to produce a particular dish. The recipe was made popular by Escoffier, a French chef who lived in the late nineteenth and early twentieth century. George Auguste Escoffier brought professionalism to the preparation of food. He standardized the white uniform and chef's hat, and he formalized the preparation of dishes through the use of recipes. He published exhaustive compilations of recipes. I have no idea if he was the greatest of all chefs, since I never ate a meal he prepared, but I expect that he was the most influential.

Recipes are a standardized way of communicating about food. Telling someone to make fried chicken leaves a lot of room for variation. Sending a particular recipe leaves less room. The recipe can be specific, with precise quantities, food temperatures, and cooking times, or it can be nonspecific, simply listing the ingredients without quantities, and giving a general description of the cooking process. The first time I encountered such a recipe, I was upset. It was an Italian recipe for a tomato soup, thickened with stale Italian bread. It has become my favorite soup, and I have come to understand the beauty of such informal recipes. They leave room for creativity, and they allow the cook to create the dish the way he or she would like it.

Highly specific recipes are useful for a restaurant. After all, the customer who comes in because he liked the Fettuccini Alfredo on his last visit might be upset if he got a different dish the next time. Of course each time it is prepared, it will be a little different, but the variation should be minimized. In addition, if the chef has a day off, a careful recipe ensures that the substitute chef will be able to prepare a passable replica of the chef's cuisine. (I still recommend that you skip the restaurant if the chef is off.)

When cooking at home I generally am not too concerned about this. I create recipes so that I can remember how I did something. The quantities are approximate. After all, the ingredients are not consistent anyway, and I try to allow for these differences. Also, my mood changes, and I may want a meal that is very spicy at one time, and the same dish in a blander version the next.

I am not recommending that you become a gourmet chef. To me, that is someone who prepares complex dishes, usually of French origin, and sometimes for very large groups. The preparation is excellent and the presentation is elegant. I have personally known only one gourmet chef. His name was Kenny Blair. Kenny was a former Hell's Angel, supposedly founder of the Oakland chapter. He had done several stints in prison. He had served in the paratroopers in World War II at the age of seventeen. After the war he moved between semi-legal pursuits and outright crime.

We met when Ken ended up coming to Synanon, a drug rehabilitation community, in about 1972, as an alternative to prison. I had come there as a "square" because I wanted to support the community and its work. Ken and I remained friends until he died of a rare lung disease in about 1987. Ken stood five feet nine inches with a good build and a handsome face. He shaved his head, which worked for his head shape. He retained a tough guy image, but spoke excellent English and was a polite and considerate man. We rode motorcycles together, and I ate many wonderful meals he prepared. Ken could cook anything, simply by reading the recipe and following it. His presentations were as elegant as anything I have ever seen, and his dishes matched the quality of any restaurant I have been to. He could cook for very large groups. But he was not creative. He needed a recipe. More than that, Ken did not like to eat, and rarely ate any of the meals he prepared. He did not like food, but he was a master technician.

If you want to cook in a restaurant, being a technician might work. After all, innovation is not really necessary, given the tens of thousands of recipes that are available.

But this book is not about cooking in a restaurant. I am neither qualified to tell you about that nor am I interested in that. If you are interested in cooking in a restaurant, I suggest that you read *Kitchen Confidential* (Bloomsbury, 2000) by Anthony Bourdain, a successful New York chef. In addition to being screamingly funny, it is an in-depth examination of what it is like to be a professional chef. He discusses the amateur-turned-pro, the dentist who is a good cook and whose friends tell him he should open a restaurant. This almost inevitably leads to ruin, since being a good cook for social occasions has little to do with running a successful restaurant. Not only does the dentist lose his shirt, but he probably loses his love of cooking as well. He also tends to lose the friends who show up for the freebies when the restaurant is new, but are nowhere to be found when the place is struggling for survival.

Bourdain notes that he loves to be invited to friend's homes for dinners. Excellent home-cooked food, he asserts, is better than restaurant food. Restaurant food is always a compromise, prepared for the average customer. When cooking for friends and family, these compromises are not necessary. You can cook it the way you think it should be cooked.

This chapter and the next are written for the person who wants to cook

INNOVATION IS THE HALLMARK OF GREAT CHEFS

While innovation is not essential to the preparation of outstanding meals, it appears to be a hallmark of great chefs. I think this is because the deep study of food and engagement in preparing it naturally leads to innovation. Innovation also adds to pride of workmanship, which motivates continued achievement. The most important innovations are not dishes but cuisines. As an example, Alice Waters is said to be the creator of California cuisine, a cooking style characterized by the use of a variety of cooking styles to take advantage of locally produced, fresh ingredients.

at home. The objective is to enable you to cook food that is appropriate to the diet, and enjoyable as well. My intention is to encourage you to stretch out, to innovate, and to make what *you* like to eat, whatever it is. My best food is always cooked for my wife and me. This is where I can be most creative, and best focus on a particular target. The more people you have to cook for, the more you have to compromise. Cooking for large groups or in a restaurant is really a different skill. It involves some of the same skill set as cooking at home, but adds a large amount of cooking logistics.

If cooking by strict adherence to a recipe is analogous to playing classical music, then my approach to cooking is analogous to jazz. It is improvisation around a theme. It is not a free-for-all. A jazz musician needs to have knowledge of the theory of music (explicit or intuitive) and a mastery of his or her instrument. The cook must understand the basic principles of the food he or she is trying to cook, and a mastery of the techniques.

These days when I want to cook something new, I use the Internet to find several recipes. I review them to understand the basics of the dish—namely, what seems to be the common thread. I then look for simplicity, availability of ingredients, and whether I would probably like it. Finally, I figure out how it might be made in a way that is compatible with a Mediterranean-style diet.

When I make the dish, I write down the recipe, as I made it, with any comments and suggestions for next time. As recipes evolve, they enter my permanent collection. Sometimes I simply invent something, although it is probably not really new. If I looked long enough, I could probably find a very similar recipe somewhere.

Even when I have worked out a recipe that I really like, there is a good chance that I will continue to vary the preparation depending on ingredients and my mood. Any recipe is just a starting point, just like a tune is a starting point for jazz.

A good example of this is the way Italians use pasta. Basically, pasta is a palate. It appears that the Italians make a sauce out of whatever source of flavor is available. This includes meat, fish, fowl, vegetables, and herbs, all in various combinations and permutations. My favorite sauces are made from flavor sources as varied as arugula, chili peppers, Brussels sprouts, and garbanzo beans.

Each variety of ethnic food that I am familiar with can serve as a basis for innovation and creativity. You begin with some basic structure, and modify it according to your particular tastes and the ingredients that are available to you. We tend to think that in a modern supermarket, we can get almost anything. However, you will generally do much better if you concentrate on ingredients that are local and fresh.

SOME BASICS OF ETHNIC CUISINES

This section will provide some simple guidelines that I use to make passable meals. An expert in any of the particular cuisines that are discussed would probably want to set me on fire for my oversimplification or even for outright errors, but this gives you a place to start if you need one.

Italian Food

Italian food is my favorite. I have already recounted some of my experiences in Italy in Chapter 1. There is a lot of good Italian food available in the United States, along with an abundance of bad Italian food. Unfortunately, decent Italian wines are expensive here, even though they are very inexpensive there.

The most fundamental ingredient of Italian cooking is olive oil. In fact, it has been speculated that the availability of olive oil is the integrating factor of a Mediterranean-style diet. The addition of olive oil to fresh vegetables makes them attractive and reduces the need for meats to create flavor. Most Italian sauces begin with a *sofrito*. This involves the sautéing of garlic, onion, and other vegetables in olive oil. Typically the vegetables that take longer to cook are put into the oil first. If you are sautéing onions, garlic, and chopped carrots, you would start with the onions and carrots. You want the carrots softened, the onions translucent, and the garlic golden, not brown. Adding tomatoes to this is the beginning of a tomato sauce. Adding ground meat would be the beginning of a *ragu,* such as Bolognese sauce.

Marcella Hazan, an Italian cookery writer, lists a number of ingredients that are particular to Italian food. These include the following:

- Herbs and spices: Basil, bay leaf, black pepper, marjoram, nutmeg, oregano, rosemary, and sage.

- Foods used for flavor: Anchovies, capers, garlic, pancetta (Italian bacon that is not smoked, therefore different from our bacon), dried porcini mushrooms, prosciutto, and radicchio.

- Cheeses: Fontina, mozzarella (especially the kind made from the milk of the water buffalo), Parmesan, ricotta, and Romano.

Many of us think first of pasta when we think of Italian food. Legend has it that pasta originated in China and was brought to Italy by the explorer Marco Polo in the fourteenth century. However, pasta can be traced back in Italy to at least 400 B.C. So pasta likely evolved independently in Europe and the Far East. The varieties of pasta are nearly endless. Both fresh and dried are good, but if you buy fresh, make sure it is freshly made, not the packaged variety. Although pasta is easy to make, I seldom do it, as it is easy to purchase good fresh pasta where I live.

Most of the meat and fish available to us can be incorporated into Italian cooking. Of course, an important feature of the food in Italy is the quality and freshness of the ingredients. There is a huge gap between the quality of their tomatoes and the ones available to me here. That's why I resort to imported, canned tomatoes for many dishes.

Asian Food

Most reasonable people would assume that if you are eating a Mediterranean-style diet, you are eating dishes from Southern Italy, the Middle East, or Northern Africa. In fact, in the original Seven Countries Study (discussed in Chapter 2), the diet of the Japanese cohort appeared as healthy as the food from the Mediterranean region. This is not surprising as the Japanese diet is low in red meat and processed foods, and high in grains and vegetables. The only problem with the Japanese diet is that many Westerners find it unattractive, and the ingredients are not widely available. Many Asian dishes adapt well to the principles of a Mediterranean-style diet. General rules are to avoid the beef and pork dishes, and use canola oil for frying. Brown rice is preferable to white rice.

I have traveled extensively in Asia. I am humbled by the variety and quality of the food. I apologize for an amateurish description of Asian cooking, but I want to convey the elegance, attractiveness, and healthiness of the food. In the first place there are countless varieties of cuisines in Asia.

In Japan I have eaten country style, traditional, teppan-yaki, sukiyaki, tempura, sushi, and shabu-shabu, each in a restaurant devoted to that particular cuisine. Each is a special art. In a tempura bar, each piece is served individually in a perfect presentation. The only Japanese food that I have had in America that compares favorably with what I have had in Japan is sushi. The Japanese have more variety, but ours is passable. Perhaps there are places in America that provide excellent representations of other Japanese styles, but I have not found them.

Most Americans have a complete misconception of Japanese food. Certainly I did. On my first trip there, in the mid-1980s, my colleague and I arrived tired after a twelve-hour fight on Japan Airlines. At least we were in business class, but the seating was tight and I had never flown that far. We got to our hotel, the Imperial, at about four o'clock in the afternoon. The Imperial, which has since been torn down, was designed by Frank Lloyd Wright and was the most prestigious hotel in Japan, if not the best. Across the street was the Imperial Palace where the emperor and his wife reside. The hotel was located in the Ginza district of Tokyo, the most westernized and by far the most expensive.

Jerry and I decided that we would have some sushi, as that seemed appropriate. We walked through the Ginza for over an hour, looking at more than 100 restaurants. Not one served sushi. We found spaghetti, hamburgers, and pizza, but no sushi. To this day, after a dozen visits, I only know one sushi restaurant in the Ginza, though I am sure there are more. However, sushi is really not the standard for Japanese food.

Finally, we entered a restaurant where the staff seemed nice and the prices were not too expensive. (It was easy in those days to pay over $100 per person for a meal in the Ginza. A continental breakfast at the Imperial was $14.) It turned out that the restaurant specialized in barbecued eel, similar to unagi in a sushi restaurant, served over a bowl of steamed rice. It was fine and the staff was wonderful. No one spoke English and the ladies giggled endlessly over the clumsy *gaijins* (foreigners).

Of the ten most memorable meals I have ever eaten, probably five were in Japan. On my first visit, our host took us to a restaurant in the Ginza.

The name of the restaurant escapes me, but I will never forget the experience. Our hosts spoke little English and there was no translator, so we smiled a lot and chuckled as though we were having a good time. This restaurant served a seven-course meal, each course having lobster as the principal ingredient. Lobster soup, a Japanese version of Lobster Thermidor, and so forth.

Toward the end, two waiters entered our private room with a very large platter that made a magnificent spectacle. The platter was about four feet by three feet. It was made to look like a seacoast scene, with rocks and seaweed. Displayed on this panorama were seven lobsters, one for each of the group, appearing as though they were in their natural habitat. (They were Pacific lobsters, without claws.) On the tail of each was a leaf of what appeared to be lettuce. On the lettuce was a scoop of something that looked a bit like potato salad. Of course our hosts would not take any food before we did, and they did not have the ability to explain in English what we should do. We figured that we should eat the "potato salad" first, as that looked the safest. My colleague Jerry reached out with his chopsticks to take some, and then it happened. His lobster moved. He turned green and I felt green. I had a revolting vision of having to dissect a living lobster to save face in front of my hosts. I began to consider what the lobster might think of me as I did this. I also began to consider immediate flight.

Fortunately, our hosts dived in and we were able to figure out that we did not need to encounter the lobster with such intimacy. The only requirement was to eat the "potato salad" which turned out to be a delicious salad made from raw lobster. The reason that the lobster was present was to prove the freshness of the dish. We later found that the name of the dish translates to "the dancing lobster." The movement of the lobster certifies that its loss of tail was quite recent. Cold-blooded beasts like lobsters have muscle activity for hours after death. I had the dish again in Taiwan, years later, without the shock.

My favorite meal of all time was in a country-style restaurant in Ibaraki, outside of Tokyo. We had been taken for a golf outing by our hosts. We had played twenty-seven holes of very expensive and very inept golf. Our caddy was a woman in her fifties with a gold front tooth. She pushed four bags on what appeared to be a modified shopping cart. Her only English was, "Nice sho." This meant nice shot. She said it to me perhaps twice in twenty-seven holes. The course had little clumps of very thin trees. If you were in the trees, as I often was, it was impossible to hit anything more than a chip shot that would not ricochet off several and stay in the thicket.

Following the golf we went to the inn and were ushered into a private room. We sat around a sand pit in which a small fire was built. While the coals were developing, we drank several bottles of the best saké I have ever tasted. When the coals were ready, a large earthenware bowl was placed over them and butter was melted in it. We were brought platters of sliced meat and fish along with bowls of several sauces. You would use your chopsticks to take a slice and sauté it briefly in the butter, then dip in the sauce and eat. Any stress was alleviated by more saké. After the meat and fish, we are served fresh vegetables to eat in the same way. Between the food and the saké, we spent several wonderful hours there.

Though many Parisians would have apoplexy at these words, it is my opinion that Hong Kong has the world's best food. The western food that I have encountered is not very good, but the varieties of Chinese food are endless and magnificent.

We find some good representations of Chinese food here, but the variety and elegance of the food found in Hong Kong and Taipei are just not there. As with Japanese food, there are many styles of Chinese cuisine. When translated to America, this has evolved into some kind of meat, fish, or fowl, lathered with gravy, and served over steamed rice. Perhaps the development of American-Chinese food was assigned to the person who developed creamed chipped beef. After about twenty visits, I have spent a total of over six months in the Chinese countries of Taiwan, Hong Kong, and China, and have never had a dish served on top of steamed rice. In fact, I never saw steamed rice at a dinner.

I have not been in Vietnam or Thailand. I have eaten both of these cooking styles in Hong Kong and find that the American versions are as good or better. Perhaps this is because so many immigrants from Southeast Asia have come to America since the Vietnam War.

The point there is that I have the deepest respect for Asian cuisine. It is, to me, the most elegant and has, by far, the greatest variety. Even if one had the skill however, it would be very difficult to reproduce it in America.

Although we have wonderful Asian markets here in San Diego, the fresh fish and the variety of fresh produce cannot be found. In addition, the huge amount of preparation time required for the more elegant styles of Chinese food, such as Cantonese, make this impractical for most home cooks and probably for all but the most expensive restaurants. However, other Chinese cuisines such as Szechwan are simpler, as are Thai and Vietnamese. My own approach is to cook westernized versions, providing healthy meals with an Asian flavor.

A tract on the basics of Asian food is beyond my capability, and would fill a book much longer than this. I will list a few things that tend to distinguish Asian food. First, Asian food is not prepared with olive oil. Use canola oil. Garlic and ginger are staples, and for some Asian cuisines, hot peppers. Soy sauce is used with or instead of salt to develop flavor, and many Chinese dishes are flavored with sesame. Scallions are usually employed rather than yellow, white, or red onions. Pungent black mushrooms and fermented black beans are another source of flavor that reduces the need for meat. Below is a list of commonly used herbs, spices, and other foods used for flavor. It is not complete, but it serves to illustrate the vast variety that is found in Asian food.

- Herbs and spices: Allspice, anise, chillies, cilantro, coriander, garlic, ginger, soy sauce, lemon grass, sesame seeds and sesame oil, and mint.

- Foods used for flavor: Citrus, fermented beans, leeks, pungent mushrooms (shiitake, black mushrooms, wood ear, oyster, etc.), miso, and scallions.

- Basic foods: All varieties of seafood, chicken and other fowl, pork, eggs, noodles, and rice; vegetables (asparagus, beans—especially black and soy, bamboo shoots, broccoli, cabbage, carrot, corn, eggplant, peas, spinach, squash, sweet potato, and water chestnuts); nuts; and fruits (apples, bananas, cherries, citrus, cucumber, mango, pear, plum, and watermelon).

- Cheeses (counterparts to): in particular, and dairy in general, are not a part of Asian cuisine. (This would appear to provide a huge and wide-open market for the National Dairy Council.) The Asian counterparts would appear to be soy products like tofu and miso. These are much healthier than cheese, as they have virtually no saturated fat.

Obviously there are substantial overlaps between Asian food and Mediterranean food. This is not surprising since, in general, some variety of the same ingredients are available in both regions. The biggest differences would seem to be the lack of olives and olive oil, tomatoes, cheese, and bread in Asian food.

Mexican Food

As mentioned earlier, my wife and I travel frequently to Ensenada, a town on the Pacific in Baja, about sixty miles south of Tijuana and just over an hour from San Diego. It is not a resort and not a border town. The main industry is tuna fishing, but there is a growing tourist business. Cruise ships dock there twice each week. More and more American ex-patriots are living there. There are several good hotels (including Coral Y Marina, Punto Morro, and Las Rosas) and at least a dozen good restaurants.

One of the things I notice on the streets is that obesity appears to be much more prevalent than in San Diego, especially among women and young boys and girls. I suspect that increasing prosperity has brought an increase in meat consumption, and goods made with sugar are everywhere. McDonald's occupies a prominent place in the center of town and does a brisk business. Ice cream appears to be very popular. Nevertheless, with a bit of care, it is not all that difficult to find a healthy meal.

Because the town is coastal, there is an emphasis on seafood. The fish tacos are good everywhere. However, most restaurants that I have been to, both in Ensenada and in nearby Puerto Villarta, usually overcook the fish. We have found a few that do not, including our favorite seafood restaurant in Ensenada, Mahi Mahi.

For most people, the idea of Mexican food brings to mind tortillas, beans, and chillies. While these are the staples, there is much more complexity. If you are interested, I suggest you read Rick Bayliss's *Mexican Kitchen* (Scribner, 1996).

The most basic flavors of Mexican cooking come from the frying of garlic, onions, chillies, often with the addition of cumin. Traditionally, the frying was done in lard, but excellent food can be cooked in canola or olive oil. Much of the taste that distinguishes one sauce from another comes from the particular chili that is used. Most of us are familiar with jalapenos and serranos, and maybe even habeneros (watch out for the heat), but there are many more including: ancho, chipotle, guajillo, pasilla, and poblano. They are often, dried, and/or roasted. Bayliss feels that the dried ancho is perhaps the most versatile chili, with "an earthy sweetness, mixed with a small dose of heat . . . "

Because I like Mexican food so much, I include this cuisine on my list, with the reservation that much of this food is not easily adapted to the Mediterranean Diet.

- Herbs and spices: Achiote seeds, all varieties of dried chillies, cilantro, coriander, cumin, epazote, garlic, marjoram, oregano, and thyme.

- Foods used for flavor: All varieties of fresh chillies, citrus (especially lime), garlic, onions, tomatillos, and dried shrimp.

- Cheeses: Chihuahua, queso fresco, and Monterey jack.

Indian Food

To me Indian food is similar to Mexican food. In fact, curry powder and chili powder are similar, containing dried chillies and cumin. I was first introduced to Indian food by a friend who had lived in Nepal while she and her husband worked for the public health service in the 1960s. They had brought back all the paraphernalia, and their former cook regularly sent spices to them. They had wonderful dinner parties where everyone used the traditional method and ate curry from tin plates with their fingers. They always had a dessert of betel nuts and provided Indian cigarettes, which looked like a dried elm leaf curled up around about six grains of tobacco.

Since that time, I have cooked versions of Indian food. I discovered very quickly that commercial curry powder is not the best way to go. I would use chili, coriander, cumin, and turmeric in proportions that suited my own taste. These were dramatically better than dishes prepared with commercial curry powder.

More about Curry

Actually, the term "curry" is a western invention. According to Brent Thompson, an expert on Indian cooking: The term curry itself isn't really used in India, except as a term appropriated by the British to generically categorize a large set of different soup and stew preparations ubiquitous in India and nearly always containing ginger, garlic, onion, turmeric, chili, and oil (except in communities which eat neither onion nor garlic, of course) and which must have seemed all the same to the British, being all yellow/red, oily, spicy/aromatic, and too pungent to taste anyway.

I have not been to India. The closest I have been was a trip to Pakistan several years ago. Until 1948, Pakistan was part of India. My company was purchasing soccer balls, made in Pakistan, which were to be delivered to our customers in Brazil and Argentina. My host in Pakistan was a wonderful and urbane fellow name Saleem, who unfortunately was killed in a fire several years ago. He was educated at the London School of Economics, and had lived in London for a number of years. He had wonderful stories, and much interesting information about Pakistan. However, the food in Pakistan was, unfortunately, unremarkable. The Indian food in London is better.

The very best Indian food that I ever had was on a brief visit to Singapore. I had dropped in from Hong Kong to visit a customer who was a Singapore citizen of Chinese heritage. He invited me to dinner and assumed I would want western food. I knew that Singapore had a large Indian population. His eyes lit up when I told him that I would like Indian food. "I know just the place," he said. We drove to an Indian section of town and he led me into a small restaurant. He told me that this was a "banana-leaf restaurant." Apparently it was traditional in this part of the world for curry to be served on a banana leaf. In this restaurant they used vinyl place mats shaped like a banana leaf.

We went to a counter to order and my host picked out several varieties. Then he said that fish head curry was a special delicacy, and asked if I would like some. I said, "Of course," and we proceeded to the table. A man was going from table to table with a wooden bucket with a shoulder strap. The bucket was filled with saffron rice, which he would kerplop onto your place mat with a large ladle. If the place sounds chaotic, it was not. It was very clean, and nicely appointed. I expect that it was a popular family restaurant, as it was full of families eating dinner.

The curries were delivered and we ladled them over our rice. My host ate with his fingers. Since that is a skill I have not acquired, or perhaps acquired and lost after babyhood, I used utensils.

The curries were wonderful and the fish head curry was the best. All were hot, but very delicate compared with any other curry I have had. To help with the heat, we were served copious quantities of thick and sweet limeade.

As we were finishing, my host looked at me and asked if I would like the eyeball of the fish, which was a special delicacy. I told him I would pass on that. He then noted that he would also pass on this opportunity. I expect that most readers will appreciate that I will also pass on providing you with a recipe for this dish.

Indian food is best cooked in canola oil, although some recipes specify clarified butter. I always substitute canola oil. Flavors are developed from garlic, onion, ginger, chillies, and spices that include cumin, coriander, and turmeric. Beef and pork are not usually a part of the cuisine for religious reasons. The favored meats are lamb, fowl, and seafood.

Many of the dishes fit quite well into the Mediterranean scheme, especially the vegetable dishes and soups.

- Herbs and spices: Cardamon, cinnamon, cloves, coriander, cumin, dried chillies, fennel seed, fenugreek, ginger, mustard seed, nutmeg, and turmeric.

- Foods used for flavor: Fresh chillies, garlic, onion, and pickled and spiced fruits and vegetables including chutney.

Other Cuisines

Almost any cuisine can be adapted to a Mediterranean-style diet, though some are easier than others. For example, the classic British diet of beef, lamb, and refined starches is a bit of a stretch, but British cuisine is not that popular anymore, even in England. Although Middle Eastern food is right on the money, I have not included it here because I don't cook it. There are guidelines for modifying recipes at the end of this chapter.

SHOPPING

One of the important truths I learned in my study of manufacturing quality was that producing a quality product was very unlikely unless you started with high-quality raw materials. While certain cuisines have been developed to deal with raw materials that are less than ideal, such as heavily spiced Indian recipes to deal with meat that is past its prime, even those cuisines are much better if you have good raw materials.

Chicken is a good case in point. When I used to buy chicken at my local supermarket, it was good about 50 percent of the time. Buying organic chickens at my local organic market is more expensive, but they are always good. The breasts are never dry unless I overcook them.

Fish is even more critical. I have not found a way to turn bad fish into a good meal. Of course, it is easy to turn good fish into a bad meal, usually by overcooking it. Buying expensive fish is not a simple answer, as the $17.95 per pound Chilean sea bass is not always good. You either need a source you absolutely trust, or you need to learn how to separate the good from the not so good. Because my trusted sources are at least a twenty-minute drive each way from me, I am working on separation. Lately I have been asking to smell the fish, and that is working very well.

Fresh vegetables are no different. If I get a russet potato from my local supermarket, it may be good. The taste of russet potatoes from my local organic market is always splendid. In fact, I think a lot of people eat insufficient amounts of vegetables because they get poor-quality vegetables. It is important to note, by the way, that I do not guarantee that your local organic market, if there is one, will be better than your local supermarket. You need to find out. In my neighborhood, the organic market is a lot better for most items.

I prefer to buy the fresh ingredients of a meal no more than a day before cooking them. Fish I almost always cook the day I buy it. I keep garlic and onions on hand, and usually have some left over leafy vegetables, a few tomatoes, and some fruit. I always have a stock of dried food, like brown rice and several varieties of beans. I stock canned tomatoes and a few other canned items, like garbanzo beans and olives. We usually have cheeses on hand, such as feta and Parmesan. Most of the fresh stuff we have on hand is because we can't use all of what we had to buy in one meal. With a family of two, a bunch of lettuce lasts two to three meals.

While we are on the topic of organic foods, I should mention that in many cases, you should buy organic for health reasons. *Consumer Reports,* which hardly encourages frivolous expenditures, recommends that you buy organic versions of the following fruits and vegetables "as often as possible": apples, bell peppers, celery, cherries, imported grapes, nectarines, peaches, pears, potatoes, red raspberries, spinach, and strawberries. They also add meat, poultry, eggs, dairy, and baby food. They believe that the significant price premium (20 to 100 percent more) is worth it to avoid pesticide residues and other harmful additives. For me, the improved flavor is worth the premium anyway.

I use about a liter of olive oil every eight to ten days. You want to buy extra-virgin, first cold press. "Extra virgin" indicates that the oil comes from the initial pressing of the olives. "Cold press" is important, as hot pressing changes the chemistry of the oil. I have found a fairly inexpensive ($7.99/liter) brand Sadaf, which I like. This is a matter of personal taste, money, and what is available in your area. I buy in liter bottles (just over a quart), as the larger cans are inconvenient.

I use an abundance of tomatoes in sauces, soups, and stew. While the recipe sometimes requires fresh tomatoes, most of my recipes use the canned variety. I have found that the imported Italian plum tomatoes have much more flavor than any of the domestic varieties I have tried. I have found an economical source and keep at least a half dozen cans in my pantry at all times. They are well worth the price premium, which is about 30 percent.

KITCHENS

I work in a lovely kitchen with a 48-inch Wolf range with six powerful burners and a grill. The kitchen has spacious granite counters, and good equipment. My son Marshall cooks in a cramped kitchen with very little counter space and a 30-inch economy electric range. Marshall turns out wonderful meals for large groups of people. The moral is that having an elegant kitchen is not essential to good cooking. A fine kitchen is like a luxury car. It does not get you there more reliably, but it can make the trip more enjoyable.

Fine kitchens are built around function, not esthetics. When we bought our present home in 1990, the kitchen was hideous. The counters were white tile with cobalt blue trim. The cabinets were falling apart, and the stove was getting rusty. Fran and I were determined to remodel.

We hired an architect to sketch some concepts for us. We were not impressed and decided to continue thinking about what we wanted. Several months later we went to a garage sale in the neighborhood and discovered that they had recently remodeled their kitchen. It was wonderfully functional, and I asked who had done it.

I contacted the person who had done the work. It turned out that he was a craftsman, a cook, and a committed surfer. He was not a kid, by the way. Like many committed surfers in Del Mar, he was well into his forties. He told me that he was not interested in doing my kitchen, since he was about to depart on a six-month surfing trip to the South Pacific. However, he said he would be happy to look at the kitchen and give me his thoughts.

We spent about an hour and I took notes. He told me never to hire an architect who was not a cook. There were a few crucial pieces of advice. The sink, dishwasher, and china cabinet should be located so that all could be reached from one position on the floor. Parallel counters should be no more than 48 inches apart, so that you could reach between them without much travel, but had sufficient space for two to work. The best move was locating the stove on the island rather than on a counter against the wall. When I cook, I am facing my guests, who tend to sit around the island. If there are no guests, or if I get bored by the ones I have, I can look out at the lovely ocean view.

The remodel was conducted at a relatively low cost, and the result is an absolutely wonderful place to work. I am sure that it has motivated me to devote more time and attention to cooking.

Barbecue Grills

Our stove has a built-in grill. I rarely use it, as cleaning it is a horrendous task. Instead I use what I consider to be the best grill you can buy. Before I bought it, my intention was to buy a good, stainless steel, propane-powered grill. My brother-in-law suggested an alternative, a grill he had owned for years: the Big Green Egg. It is green and shaped like an egg, about 20 inches in diameter and 30 inches tall. It is constructed of a ceramic material about $3/4$ inches thick. The top section hinges up to expose the grill. It has adjustable vents on the top and bottom to control the airflow, and therefore the temperature. It runs on natural wood charcoal, which I light with an electric starter. The natural wood charcoal burns faster and makes very little ash. It takes approximately fifteen minutes to reach grilling temperature, as measured by a temperature gauge on the grill. The temperature can be adjusted from 250°F to 700°F by using the vents. It holds accurately to within 5°F to 10°F. Most grilling is done between 350°F and 500°F. Because the lid is closed and the airflow is regulated, there are no flames to burn the meat or vegetables.

I grill whole chickens by butterflying them and grilling at 375°F for approximately forty-five minutes, turning once. These are the best I have ever made. There is a tendency to burn the skin on a conventional grill, especially when cooking in this amount of time.

When the cooking is finished, you close the vents and the fire goes out, preserving most of the charcoal for the next meal.

We use this grill for all barbecuing, including turkeys at Thanksgiving.

There are a number of well-made charcoal and gas grills that provide an alternative. I have owned both types and neither is more convenient than the Egg. Gas grills require a lot of cleaning and the grills that use charcoal briquettes take much longer to light. Neither will hold a steady temperature like the Egg. However, you can make excellent food with either type. My one caveat is never to use charcoal lighter fluid, unless you like the way it tastes.

Equipment

The mechanical essentials are a blender, and a hand blender. A stand mixer and a food processor are also nice. I use the food processor regularly to make hummus. I rarely use the stand blender, but it is very attractive. I love good knives but you really only need a chef's knife, a slicing knife, and a smaller paring knife or boning knife. I have a lot more, including a sushi knife, which is beveled on only one side of the edge. I rarely use anything but one of the three basics.

For pans, you need at least one fry pan, a saucepan, and one or two stockpots, plus a non-stick fry pan. I do not like nonstick pans for most cooking, but they are essential for eggs and for fried rice. One of my most frequently used pans is a deep skillet with a lid. These are frequently called chicken frying pans and are hard to find. Mine is 11 inches in diameter and 4 inches deep in stainless steel. I use it for most pasta sauces, and many vegetable dishes. It is deep enough to cook dishes that have liquid.

I recommend stainless steel pans with an aluminum sandwich for heat distribution. The best I have used are All-Clad, but they are expensive. The cheaper pans tend to have the aluminum sandwich only on the bottom and food tends to burn on the sides. On the All-Clad pans, the sandwich extends part way up the side. I don't like aluminum pans because the aluminum is likely to leach into your food. This is especially likely with acidic dishes like tomato sauces. While anodized aluminum will not leach, the anodizing layer is quite thin and will eventually wear off.

Because brown rice is a staple in the Laguna Beach Diet, I recommend a rice cooker. If you get a cheaper one, you will have to do a bit of trial and error to get the right amount of water, as brown rice requires more than the white rice that the cooker was designed for. My son uses an inexpensive model and it works well. Some of the more expensive models have a setting for brown rice. I have an expensive one, but it does not have a brown-rice setting. I add a bit more water and it works beautifully. Whether you have an inexpensive one or a luxury model, you simply add rice and water and turn it on. It will cook the rice and keep it warm until you are ready to eat.

If you like to eat beans, I recommend a pressure cooker for when you do not have time to soak and prepare dried beans. My son turned me on to this. He lived in Brazil for about six months with his Brazilian soon-to-be bride. Brazilians eat a lot of beans and he says every Brazilian (who has a kitchen) uses a pressure cooker. You can cook dried pinto beans in about thirty minutes from start to finish. (Much of this time is rinsing the beans and getting the water to boil. Cooking time is around twenty-five minutes.) My pressure cooker is a Fagor. It was relatively inexpensive and works well.

Another tool that is convenient is a steamer. My wife bought a Black & Decker steamer at a garage sale for five dollars. (You can probably get a new one for less than forty dollars.) It is great for broccoli, cauliflower, green beans, and even potatoes. Again, you put in the vegetables and water and hit the switch. Serve the veggies with a little salt and they are wonderful—assuming you started with good produce.

COOKBOOKS AND RECIPES

When I want a recipe, I usually search online and find several, and create my own recipe based on what ingredients I have and what I think will work best for my taste. I use cookbooks for theory. The four that are most important to me, in order, are: *Essentials of Classic Italian Cooking* (Knopf, 1992) by Marcella Hazan, *Mexican Kitchen* (Scribner, 1996) by Rick Bayless, *Theory and Practice of Good Cooking* (Knopf, 1984) by James Beard, and *Roasting: A Simple Art* (Morrow, 1995) by Barbara Kafka. I am sure that there are hundreds of other good cookbooks, but these are the ones I know.

I am not looking for collections of recipes. Hazan explains the "essentials" of Italian cooking quite well and, in my opinion, is a must read for those aspiring to Italian cooking. Bayliss is clearly a student of Mexican cooking, and operates two outstanding Mexican restaurants in Chicago, Frontera Grill and Topolobampa. His book explains the theory behind the recipes. Beard, now deceased, was often called "the dean of American cooking." His book is a fundamental reference. Kafka's book is a very creative take on roasting. You may come up with your own reference set, although I recommend that everyone should include the Hazan book. If you do not like Mexican food, for example, you can skip the Bayless book. But what is important is that you learn the theory behind the food you intend to cook. What are the basic ingredients and processes of the cuisine? If you know this, you can improvise. Thus you will be able to make many of the dishes you like, and stay within the principles of the Laguna Beach Diet. If you do not know this, you either have to slavishly follow recipes, or deduce the theory from the recipes.

Most of the Asian cookbooks I have tried have been too complex for my taste. Many classical Chinese and Japanese dishes are quite intricate, require more preparation time than I want to spend, and use ingredients that are difficult to obtain. However, this does not diminish my enthusiasm for Asian dishes. I simply need to find relatively simple ones. The most useful cookbook that I have found for healthy Asian food is *A Spoonful of Ginger* (Knopf, 1999) by Nina Simonds. Most of the recipes are relatively simple and the ingredients are not too esoteric.

While I have not found the ultimate Indian cookbook, *Curries Without Worries* (Warner, 1996) by Sudha Koul is a simple and easy to follow book with some very good recipes.

I frequently modify recipes to make them more appropriate to the Laguna Beach Diet. There are many ways to do this, and still get an acceptable result:

• Butter: You can often use olive oil instead of butter. An alternative to this is to use a small amount of butter along with olive oil. You can also try a healthy margarine, such as Smart Balance as a substitute, though I have usually not been satisfied with this. Some things will just not work without butter. I tend to avoid them, but you can certainly make them occasionally.

• Cream: Cream is used for flavor and texture, and appears to be indispensable in some sauces. In many soups I find that low-fat yogurt is a passable substitute.

• Red meat: Ground turkey and turkey sausage are an acceptable lower fat substitute for ground beef in many recipes. I was surprised to discover that I could make excellent Bolognese sauce with ground turkey. I prefer turkey meatloaf, and am very happy with turkey burgers. However, remember that even ground turkey has a significant amount of saturated fat, so you can't eat unlimited amounts. When products like sausage, bacon, and pancetta are used for the flavor they add, I often reduce the amounts. This may be a trial and error process for you at first.

• Whole grains: Whenever possible, I substitute whole grains for refined products. I use brown rice rather than white rice, except in risotto, where

I can't get it to work. I use whole-wheat flour instead of refined flour, and often use whole-wheat pasta. This works pretty well with a robust sauce, but less well for a delicate sauce.

The more general point is that as you learn to cook, you can find many opportunities to create dishes you like that are very consistent with the Laguna Beach Diet.

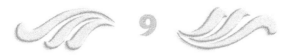

9

Recipes

THE FOLLOWING RECIPES ARE THINGS that I cook and enjoy. Some are completely original, some are traditional dishes, and some are modifications of dishes to enable them to fit the diet. The basic cuisines of the Laguna Beach Diet—Mediterranean, Asian, and Mexican—are represented. They are included partly for the reader to cook, and partly to give the reader an idea of how to create more recipes. Remember, that I am not a gourmet chef, and that this is not really a cookbook. Keeping that in mind, I hope this chapter will help you to enjoy the Laguna Beach Diet.

SOUPS AND STEWS

Chicken Stew with Leeks

This is a bit unusual, but the combination of chicken, leeks, and lemon really works.

YIELD: SERVES 4–6

2–3 tablespoons extra-virgin olive oil

2 pounds boneless skinless chicken thighs, cut in half

salt and pepper, to taste

4 medium carrots, coarsely chopped

4 ribs celery, chopped

4 medium leeks, white part only, chopped

3 parsnips, peeled and chopped

6 cloves garlic, peeled and finely chopped

1 teaspoon dried thyme

1 teaspoon dried tarragon

½ cup red wine

4–8 cups chicken stock (preferably homemade)

2 tablespoons lemon juice

½ cup dried orzo or other small pasta

Parmesan cheese, grated

loaf of coarse Italian bread

In a large pot, heat the oil and brown the chicken pieces over medium heat, adding salt and pepper. When the chicken is lightly browned, add the vegetables and garlic and sauté for about 10 minutes over medium heat, stirring frequently. Next add the thyme and tarragon. Then season with more salt and pepper. Add the red wine. Deglaze the pot and reduce the wine for about 5 minutes. Add the lemon juice and enough stock to cover. Bring to a boil, then reduce heat and simmer for about 15 to 30 minutes until the chicken and vegetables are cooked to your taste. Adjust for salt, then add the pasta, more stock if necessary, and cook until done.

Serve with grated Parmesan cheese and chunks of coarse Italian bread on the side.

Eggplant Stew with Sausage and Garbanzo Beans

This is a hearty dish, good even without the sausage.

YIELD: SERVES 4

2 tablespoons extra-virgin olive oil

1–2 links of turkey sausage, cut into 1-inch pieces (optional)

1 medium onion, coarsely chopped

3 garlic cloves, finely chopped

1 red, yellow, or orange bell pepper, seeded, deveined, and chopped

$\frac{1}{2}$ jalapeno chili, finely chopped

$\frac{1}{2}$ teaspoon chili powder

1 tablespoon cinnamon

2 tablespoons ground cumin

$\frac{1}{2}$ teaspoon salt

1 large eggplant, diced into 1-inch pieces

1 can (14-ounces) garbanzo beans, drained and rinsed

1 can (14-ounces) chopped tomatoes

1 cup chicken stock (preferably homemade)

salt and pepper, to taste

Heat oil in a large, heavy bottom skillet or large pot. Add sausage, if desired, and cook until it begins to brown. Add onion, garlic, jalapeno, bell pepper, spices, and $\frac{1}{2}$ teaspoon of salt. Stir well and cook over medium heat until onions are translucent. Add eggplant, garbanzo beans, tomatoes, and stock. Bring to a boil. Cover, then reduce heat and simmer for about 45 minutes, stirring occasionally, until eggplant is tender. Add salt and pepper to taste.

Med Chili

*I love chili and especially the recipes of Rick Bayliss.
This is a bit simpler and still good. There are many things you
can add. Once I added dried Chinese black mushrooms about 15
minutes before serving so that they were still a bit crunchy.
Everybody loved it. One of my friends keeps asking for it again
and again. I could call it "Chinese chili." This particular version
is based on ingredients that fit well into a Mediterranean Diet.
It tastes like chili with a slight Italian flair.*

YIELD: SERVES 8

1½ cups dried Great Northern white beans

2–3 tablespoons extra-virgin olive oil

1 medium onion, chopped

4–6 cloves garlic, minced

2 ribs celery, chopped

1 medium carrot, diced

1 red bell pepper, seeded, deveined, and diced.

1 pound ground turkey (or ½ pound ground breast and
½ pound of whole ground turkey)

½ teaspoon pepper, freshly ground

2 tablespoons chili powder, or to taste

1 tablespoon ground cumin

½ cup dry white wine

1 can (28-ounces) peeled plum tomatoes with their juices,
cut into 1-inch pieces (preferably imported Italian tomatoes)

1–2 teaspoons sugar, to taste

salt and pepper, to taste

Beans. Soak the beans in water for at least 6 hours, or overnight. Quick soaking can be done by boiling the beans in water for 2 to 3 minutes and then removing from heat, covering, and soaking for 2 hours.

After soaking, drain and rinse beans several times. Cover with 2 inches of water, bring to a boil and simmer for 30 to 90 minutes until done. Stir occasionally. Add water if necessary. The beans are done when they can be easily crushed between thumb and forefinger. Do not add salt until the beans are nearly cooked. Then start with $1/2$ teaspoon and adjust to taste. Reserve the beans and their water until ready to add to the chili.

Chili. While the beans are cooking, heat the olive oil in a large pot and sauté the onion, garlic, celery, carrot, and bell pepper for 4 to 5 minutes, until the onions begin to soften. Add the meat and generously salt it. Add approximately $1/2$ teaspoon of freshly ground pepper. Add the chili powder and cumin. Stir frequently to crumble the meat and mix in the spices. Cook until the vegetables are soft and the meat is no longer red (about 20 minutes). Add the wine and reduce for 5 minutes. Add the tomatoes with their juices, and stir well. Simmer slowly, uncovered for 1 to 2 hours, stirring occasionally. Test for salt and add sugar to adjust for the acidity of the tomatoes. I generally use about 1 to 2 teaspoons of sugar. If the sauce seems dry, add water as necessary. Then add the beans and adjust for salt. Add the reserved cooking water from the beans if necessary to cover the beans and vegetables in the chili.

Serve with warm corn tortillas or with tortilla chips. If you use chips be careful to ensure that they were cooked in healthy oil with no saturated fat or trans fat.

Mulligatawny Stew

The word Mulligatawny derives from the Indian word for pepper
water. It appears to have been invented by the Indians for the
British Raj. Because of the name, my wife, whose mother was
born in Ireland, believes that it is an Irish dish. She asks for it
frequently. While many call it a soup, to me it is a stew. We eat
it as a main dish served over rice. The recipe below should be
viewed as a starting point. You can use different meats and
vegetables. Most recently, I used chicken sausage and added
several kinds of summer squash that I had on hand.

YIELD: SERVES 4

2 tablespoons extra-virgin olive oil

1 pound boneless, skinless chicken thighs, cut into 1-inch pieces

2 ribs celery, chopped

2 carrots, chopped

1 medium onion, coarsely chopped

$\frac{1}{2}$ small head of cauliflower (about 1$\frac{1}{2}$ cups,
separated into 1-inch florets)

$\frac{1}{2}$–1 jalapeno chili, to taste

4 cloves garlic, finely chopped

salt and pepper, to taste

1–2 tablespoons curry powder, to taste

1 tablespoon ground cumin

4 cups chicken stock (preferably homemade)

$\frac{1}{2}$ cup lentils

1 teaspoon sugar

$\frac{1}{2}$ cup low-fat yogurt

2 to 3 cups brown rice, cooked

additional yogurt, and chutney and/or Indian pickled vegetables, for garnish

Heat olive oil in a large, heavy bottomed pot. Add the chicken, celery, carrots, onion, cauliflower, jalapeno, and garlic. Add salt and pepper to taste. Sauté, stirring frequently, until the onion is translucent. Stir in the curry powder and cumin and cook for several minutes. Pour in the stock and add the lentils and sugar. Bring to a boil. Reduce heat and simmer for 30 to 60 minutes. Adjust for salt, pepper, and sugar. Stir in the yogurt about 5 minutes prior to serving. Serve in individual bowls over rice. Garnish with more yogurt, chutney, and/or Indian pickled vegetables.

Stuffed Cabbage Pot

This is a recipe from Nina Simonds' A Spoonful of Ginger (Knopf, 1999). She modified it from the traditional recipe, which uses pork. She recommends it for cool weather, but I love it in San Diego where the weather is never really cool. The soup reheats beautifully. (Reprinted with permission from author.)

YIELD: SERVES 4

Soup

1 medium head Napa cabbage, about 1/2–3/4 pounds

1 teaspoons canola oil

4 cloves garlic, peeled and smashed lightly with the flat side of a knife

1/3 cup rice wine or saké

5 cups chicken stock (preferably homemade)

Meatballs

1 pound ground turkey

6 dried Chinese black mushrooms, softened in hot water for 20 minutes, stems removed, and caps finely chopped

2 tablespoons soy sauce

3/4 teaspoon salt

2 tablespoons minced scallions, white part only

1½ tablespoons fresh ginger, minced

2 tablespoons soy sauce

2 tablespoons rice wine or saké

1½ teaspoons toasted sesame oil

½ teaspoon freshly ground black pepper

1 tablespoon cornstarch

1 teaspoon canola oil

Soup. To make the soup, cut away the stem of the cabbage and discard. Remove and reserve four of the outermost leaves. Cut the remaining cabbage in half and cut the leaves into 2-inch squares, separating the leafy sections from the stem pieces. Set aside in two bowls.

In a Dutch oven or flameproof covered casserole, add 1 teaspoon of the oil and heat until hot, about 30 seconds. Add the garlic cloves and tougher cabbage sections and stir-fry for a minute over medium-high heat. Add the rice wine or saké and toss lightly; cover and cook for 1½ minutes. Uncover and add the remaining cabbage pieces and the chicken stock. Partially cover and once the soup reaches a boil, uncover, lower the heat, and simmer for 30 minutes.

Meatballs. Make the meatballs while the soup is cooking. Mix all of the meatball ingredients in a bowl. Use your hands to combine the ingredients evenly, then shape into four oval balls.

Preheat the oven to 350°F. Heat a wok or skillet, add the canola oil, and heat until very hot. Place the meatballs in the pan and sear until golden over high heat. Then turn over and sear the other side.

Remove the meatballs with a slotted spoon and place in the center of the cabbage soup. Cover with the four reserved leaves. Replace the lid and put the pot in the middle shelf of the oven. Bake for 45 minutes. Add the soy sauce and salt to taste and ladle into soup bowls. Serve immediately.

Nip and Nip Soup

*My wife and I were served this dish in a bed and breakfast in
the Lake District in the north of England. The cook was not
present, so I had to figure out how to make it. I decided she
used parsnips and turnips. Since the cook was English,
I am sure that she made hers with heavy cream,
but this one is excellent without it.*

YIELD: SERVES 4–6

1 tablespoon extra-virgin olive oil

1 medium onion, chopped

½–1 jalapeno chili, chopped

2 ribs celery, chopped

6 cups chicken stock (preferably homemade)

4 medium parsnips, peeled and cut into several pieces

3 medium turnips, peeled and quartered

¼ teaspoon white pepper

¼ teaspoon nutmeg

salt, to taste

1 cup low-fat yogurt, for garnish

Heat oil in a large heavy-bottomed pot. Add onion, jalapeno, and celery.
Sauté until soft. Add stock, parsnips, and turnips, then bring to boil. Add
white pepper and nutmeg. Cook until the parsnips and turnips begin to fall
apart. Purée. The simplest method is to use a hand blender to purée the
soup while in the pot. Add salt to taste. Serve with a couple of tablespoons
of yogurt in each bowl as a garnish.

Tomato and Bread Soup

The bread is important. You want a coarse bread so that it does not create lumps in the soup. I leave the crust on.

YIELD: SERVES 6–8

3 tablespoons extra-virgin olive oil, plus more for serving

½ medium onion, chopped

½–1 jalapeno chili, finely chopped

6 garlic cloves, peeled and finely chopped

1 28-ounce can of plum tomatoes with their juices
(preferably imported Italian tomatoes)

5 fresh basil leaves, shredded

4 cups chicken stock (preferably homemade)

5 slices coarse Italian bread, cut ½ inch thick, and toasted

salt and pepper, to taste

1 teaspoon sugar or more to taste

In a deep, heavy pot heat the olive oil over medium heat. Sauté the onions, jalapeno, and garlic until the onions are translucent. Add the tomatoes, their juices, and the basil to the pot. Bring to a boil, stirring occasionally. Lower heat and simmer, stirring occasionally. Cook for 1 to 2 hours, until the tomatoes begin to break down. Add the stock and the bread slices, and simmer another hour, stirring occasionally. Adjust salt, and add sugar to taste, starting with about 1 teaspoon. Purée the soup in the pot with a wand blender, and serve.

MEAT AND FISH DISHES

Chicken Stir-Fry

*You can vary the vegetables in this simple dish,
according to what you have and what you like.
Adding about a teaspoon of minced ginger when
you add the onions and garlic is good too.*

YIELD: SERVES 4

3 tablespoons soy sauce

2 tablespoons dry sherry

1 tablespoon cornstarch

1 tablespoon sugar

$\frac{1}{2}$ cup water

2 tablespoons canola oil

$1\frac{1}{2}$ pounds boneless skinless half breasts
or thighs in $\frac{3}{4}$-inch dice

3 cloves garlic, peeled and finely chopped

$1\frac{1}{2}$ cups broccoli, cut into bite-size pieces

2 cups cauliflower, separated into 1-inch florets

1 small onion, chopped

1 carrot, cut into $1\frac{1}{2}$-inch lengths
and then sliced into thin strips

1 bell pepper, seeded, veined and diced in $\frac{3}{4}$-inch pieces

2–3 cups brown rice, cooked

Combine soy sauce, dry sherry, cornstarch, sugar, and water and set aside.
Heat the oil in a large skillet over medium-high heat. Add the chicken and
cook until nearly done, tossing frequently. Remove chicken and add the
garlic and vegetables to the skillet. Cook until done, tossing frequently.

Return the chicken and add soy sauce mixture. Cook until the sauce begins to thicken. Serve over brown rice.

Note: A challenge is to get all of the ingredients done to the proper degree. First, this depends on how you like them, from al dente to well done. Cooking time depends on the density of the vegetables and the size of the pieces. Many recipes suggest cooking the chicken first then removing it to cook the vegetables. The chicken is returned when you add the sauce. But, you can simply add the vegetables before the chicken is done. This makes the timing more difficult, however.

Pan-Roasted Chicken

The quality of the chicken is critical here. Buy the best you can, such as free-range, organic, if possible.

YIELD: SERVES 4

1 tablespoon extra-virgin olive oil

1 bell pepper, seeded, deveined,
and chopped in 1-inch pieces

½–1 small jalapeno chili, finely chopped
(optional)

2 ribs celery, chopped

1 medium onion, chopped

4 boneless, skinless half-chicken breasts

Preheat oven to 350°F. Heat oil over medium heat in heavy, oven-safe frying pan. Add bell pepper, jalapeno (if using), celery, and onion to pan and sauté until they begin to soften. Add chicken and brown it on one side for about 5 minutes. Turn chicken over and put pan in the oven. Roast in the oven until done, about 7 to 12 minutes, depending on the thickness of the breasts. Serve covered with the sautéed vegetables.

Pan-Roasted Fish

The quality of the fish is critical. If you do not have absolute trust in the merchant, smell the fish before you buy it.

YIELD: SERVES 4

1 tablespoon extra-virgin olive oil

3 cloves garlic, finely chopped

1½ pounds fresh fish fillets, such as tilapia, catfish, halibut, cod, mahi-mahi, or other mild-tasting fish

salt and pepper, to taste

lemon slices, for garnish

Preheat oven to 350°F. Heat oil over medium heat in heavy, oven-safe frying pan. Sauté the garlic for 2 minutes. Add fish, sprinkle with salt and pepper, and cook on one side, about 3 to 6 minutes, depending on thickness. If the fillet has skin, cook the skin side down first and when you turn it over, you can easily remove the skin. Turn fillets over and put pan in the oven. Roast in the oven until done, about 5 to 10 minutes, depending on the thickness. You are trying to produce a moist fillet that just begins to flake. With experience you will learn to judge the timing. I look at the edges and turn when I see them begin to cook. Serve immediately, with lemon slices on the side.

Fish Tacos

This is really a combination of two recipes, pan-roasted fish and Asian slaw. When the fish is of quality and cooked properly, and when the tortillas are good, these are as delicious as any fish tacos I have had in Baja. In Baja, the fresh tortillas are superior, but my fish and slaw are better.

YIELD: MAKES 8–12 TACOS

1 lb fresh fish fillets such as tilapia, catfish, halibut, cod, mahi-mahi

1 egg, beaten lightly

½ cup breadcrumbs

3 cups Asian Slaw (for recipe see page 183)

12 corn tortillas, warmed

hot sauce, to taste

Prepare the Asian slaw ahead of time and chill.

Preheat oven to 350°F. Dredge the fillets in the egg, then coat with breadcrumbs. Prepare fish according to the method for Pan-Roasted Fish on page 153. Place cooked fish on a platter. I let the diners cut pieces of fish and assemble the tacos with fish and slaw. Those who want can add hot sauce.

Hint: The best way to warm tortillas is in a plastic container made for this. Place in the container, microwave for 30 to 60 seconds, remove, then cover.

Turkey Burgers

*Having grown up in the United States, I still have an attraction
to hamburgers. These work for me.*

YIELD: MAKES 4 BURGERS

1 pound ground turkey

1–2 tablespoons extra-virgin olive oil

½ cup red onion, finely chopped

3 cloves garlic, minced

½ cup breadcrumbs (Panko-style preferred)

1 tablespoon ground cumin

1 teaspoon salt

1 tablespoon Worcestershire sauce

4 whole-grain buns

tomato, red onion, avocado, feta cheese,
and lettuce, sliced for garnish

Combine the first eight ingredients in a bowl and mix thoroughly. Make patties of a size and thickness to your taste. I usually make four from a pound. If you have time, chill in refrigerator for at least 1 hour. Grill over medium-high heat.

Serve on a whole-grain bun. On the side, offer sliced tomatoes, sliced red onion, sliced avocado, sliced feta cheese, lettuce, mustard, and ketchup.

Turkey Meatloaf

This is a robust recipe. You can put in the ingredients you want and get a good result. I rarely make it the same way twice.

YIELD: SERVES 4

1 tablespoon extra-virgin olive oil

½ cup onion, finely chopped

½–1 jalapeno chili, finely chopped (optional)

2 pounds ground turkey

¾ cup breadcrumbs

½ cup grated carrot

½ cup sweet pickle relish

½ cup mustard

½ cup sweet chili sauce*

½ teaspoon salt

Preheat oven to 350°F. Heat oil over medium heat in frying pan. Sauté the onion and jalapeno (if using) until they begin to soften. Turn into a large bowl and mix well with the turkey, breadcrumbs, carrot, relish, mustard, sweet chili sauce, and salt. Mold into a non-stick loaf pan. Bake for 45 minutes. Pour off oil and turn meatloaf out onto a baking sheet and bake for another 30 minutes.

Variation: Substitute either ¾ cup of matzo farfel or ¾ cup oatmeal soaked for 30 minutes in ½ cup of milk for the breadcrumbs.

*A Thai-style chili sauce available in many large supermarkets or in Asian markets. Ketchup can be substituted.

BEAN AND GRAIN DISHES

Really Good Beans

*There are many ways to cook beans. This is one I really like.
Rather than soaking overnight, I begin the soak in the morning
and then cook them for supper.*

YIELD: SERVES 8–10

3 tablespoons extra-virgin olive oil

4 ounces hot Italian turkey sausage, cut into ¾ sections

1 large onion, chopped

3 ribs celery, chopped

1 large carrot, chopped

2 poblano chillies, seeded, veined, and chopped
(if unavailable substitute Anaheims)

6 cloves garlic, peeled and crushed

4 cups dried red kidney beans,
soaked for at least 8 hours and rinsed

1 bunch bok choy, Swiss chard, or kale, chopped

salt and pepper, to taste

Heat the olive oil in a large pot over medium-high heat and add the
sausage. When it begins to brown, add the vegetables (except for the
greens) and garlic. Continue to cook, stirring frequently. When the onions,
carrots, and celery begin to soften, add the beans and cover with water to
about 1 inch above the beans. Bring to a boil, stirring frequently. Reduce
heat and simmer slowly until beans are done, stirring occasionally. This will
take 30 to 90 minutes. Add water if the level goes below the beans, but at
the end you want the liquid at about the level of the beans. When the
beans are done, add the greens, and salt and pepper to taste.

Cajun Red Beans

Combined with brown rice, this makes a complete meal.

YIELD: SERVES 4–6

1–2 tablespoons extra-virgin olive oil

6 ounces Andouille sausage (may substitute Italian
turkey sausage), cut into ½-inch slices

½ medium onion, chopped

4–6 cloves garlic, finely chopped

1 large carrot, diced into ½-inch pieces

1 cup collard greens, kale, or Swiss chard, shredded

2 cups dried red beans, soaked at least 8 hours then rinsed

1 12-ounce can crushed tomatoes,
preferably imported Italian tomatoes

1 teaspoon Cajun Creole seasoning (if unavailable
substitute ½ teaspoon cayenne pepper)

salt, pepper, and sugar, to taste

2 to 3 cups brown rice, cooked

Heat olive oil in a pot and add sausage, onion, garlic, and carrot. When
onion begins to soften, add the beans, tomatoes, and seasoning. Salt and
pepper to taste. Add enough water to cover by 1 inch and bring to a boil,
stirring occasionally. Lower heat and simmer uncovered until the beans are
done, 30 to 90 minutes. Add the shredded greens. Then add salt, pepper,
and sugar to taste. Serve over brown rice.

Note: You can also quick soak the beans by boiling them in water for 2 to 3
minutes and then removing from heat, covering, and soaking for 2 hours.
Then follow the recipe for dried beans.

Variation: You may substitute two 12-ounce cans of red beans for the dried
beans. Rinse and drain well. Heat olive oil in a pot and add sausage, onion,

garlic, and carrot. When onion begins to soften, add the tomatoes, seasoning, and 1 cup water. Bring to a boil and simmer for 25 minutes. Add the beans and salt, pepper, and sugar to taste. If necessary, add enough water to cover the beans. Simmer until the beans are warm, add the shredded greens, and serve over brown rice.

Lima Beans

My wife brought home some giant, organic, dried Lima beans from a local farmers' market and we discovered that this is a wonderful dish with a unique flavor. Although the giant Limas were best, baby Limas work well also.

YIELD: SERVES 4

1½ tablespoons extra-virgin olive oil

½ medium onion, chopped

3 cloves garlic, finely chopped

½ teaspoon crushed, dried red chillies (optional)

1 pound dried Lima beans, soaked for at least 8 hours

½ teaspoon salt

salt and pepper, to taste

In a pot, heat the oil and sauté the onions, garlic, and chillies (if using) until the onions are translucent. Add the beans and enough water to cover by about 1 inch. Add ½ teaspoon of salt and bring to a boil, stirring occasionally. Reduce heat to a simmer and cook until the beans are done. This can range from 30 to 90 minutes. Stir occasionally and add water to cover beans as necessary. At the end, you don't want a lot of excess water. The result will be a thick, starchy soup. Test for salt and pepper, and serve.

Risotto

This is made by frying the rice a bit in hot oil and then slowly adding hot liquid until the rice is done. It works best with Arborio rice, but other types of white rice may be substituted. My son claims that he can do it with brown rice, but it does not work for me. You can add many things to the dish such as sausage, shrimp, Brussels sprouts, mushrooms, or almost anything that you think would taste good. If using sausage, cook it with the onions and garlic. If using shrimp, boil it a bit in the stock and add at the end so it is not overcooked.

YIELD: SERVES 4

2 tablespoons extra-virgin olive oil

$\frac{1}{2}$ medium onion, finely chopped

3 cloves garlic, finely chopped

2 cups Arborio rice

black pepper, freshly ground, to taste

6 cups chicken stock (preferably homemade), simmering

salt and pepper, to taste

Parmesan cheese, grated

In a pot, heat the oil and fry the onions and garlic until the onions are translucent. Add the rice and some black pepper. Stir well to coat all of the rice. Add about $\frac{1}{2}$ cup of the hot stock and stir. As the stock is absorbed, add $\frac{1}{2}$ cup more, continuing to stir from time to time. Continue until the rice is done to your taste, about 20 to 30 minutes. Test for salt, although the stock will likely provide enough. Serve with grated Parmesan cheese.

Fried Rice

You can use just about any vegetables you want in this.
Carrots, bell peppers, zucchini, eggplant, and mushrooms are
all tasty additions. You can use shrimp instead of chicken, or a
bit of turkey sausage. Use a nonstick pan or the rice will stick,
making cooking difficult and cleaning nearly impossible.

YIELD: SERVES 4–6

2 tablespoons extra-virgin olive oil

Boneless, skinless chicken breast in ¾-inch dice (optional)

½–1 jalapeno chili, finely chopped

½ onion, finely chopped

2 ribs celery, finely chopped

4–6 cloves garlic, finely chopped

4 cups cooked brown rice, cooked and cooled

1 12-ounce can garbanzo beans, rinsed and drained

1 teaspoon sesame oil

1 tablespoon soy sauce

⅓ cup scallions, finely chopped

½ cup peanuts

Prepare rice ahead and store in the refrigerator long enough to cool. Heat olive oil in a nonstick pan. Add chicken or shrimp (if using) and cook until nearly cooked, about 3 to 4 minutes, tossing frequently. Then add jalapeno, onion, celery, and garlic. Cook until onion is transparent, about 3 to 4 minutes, continuing to toss frequently. Add cooled rice, garbanzos, sesame oil, and soy sauce, and cook until warmed through. Toss to break up chunks and mix thoroughly. Test for salt. Garnish with scallions and peanuts, and serve.

PASTA DISHES

Lasagna with Eggplant

This takes some time to make. I serve it at parties. Olives, crumbled Italian turkey sausage, and mushrooms all make good additions to the sauce, depending on your taste.

YIELD: SERVES 6–8

1 medium eggplant, sliced lengthways about $\frac{1}{4}$ inch thick

10 dried lasagne noodles

3 cups tomato sauce (use a good commercial sauce or make one)

Approximately $\frac{1}{2}$ cup extra-virgin olive oil

1 pound part-skim ricotta cheese

$\frac{1}{2}$ pound mozzarella cheese

$\frac{1}{2}$ cup Parmesan cheese, grated

Preheat the oven to 375°F. Heat about 2 tablespoon of the olive oil in a skillet (preferably nonstick) and sauté the sliced eggplant. It will soak up a lot of oil, so add more as needed to prevent sticking. Sauté each slice until cooked through and golden. Cool and drain on paper towels.

Cook the lasagna noodles as directed on the package, drain, and cool.

Assemble the lasagna in a 9-inch by 11-inch baking dish. Put some sauce in the bottom. Cover with a layer of pasta. Cover this with a thin layer of sauce, and some of the ricotta and mozzarella. Use eggplant slices instead of pasta for the next layer. Continue alternating with layers of eggplant and pasta, covering each with the sauce and cheeses. Use pasta for the top layer, covered with the sauce and cheeses. I make either three or five layers.

Bake for 30 minutes, then top with the Parmesan and bake 10 more minutes.

Lasagna with Sweet Potato Sauce

My wife suggested a dish like this and we hit a home run.

YIELD: SERVES 4–6

3 medium sweet potatoes (garnet yams recommended)

1–2 tablespoons extra virgin olive oil

1 medium onion, chopped

2 ribs celery, chopped

½–1 jalapeno chili, finely chopped

¾ pound ground turkey

½ teaspoon salt

¼ teaspoon pepper

1 tablespoon ground cumin

dash of cayenne pepper (optional)

1–2 cups chicken stock (canned or homemade)

9–12 dried lasagna noodles

1 pound part-skim ricotta cheese

1 cup grated Parmesan cheese

Heat oven to 375°F. Bake the sweet potatoes until very soft, about 1 hour and 15 minutes. Remove from oven and allow to cool.

Heat olive oil in a saucepan and cook onion, celery, and jalapeno, until onions are translucent. Add turkey, salt, pepper, cumin and cayenne (if using). Continue to cook, breaking up the turkey into small chunks. When the turkey loses its red color, lower the heat and add the sweet potatoes. I slice them lengthwise and scoop out chunks of the flesh with a teaspoon. Since you want to form a sauce, you do not want large chunks. Then add about 1 cup of the stock. Cook and stir until a sauce forms, adding more stock if necessary. You do not want the sauce too thin, as it needs to sit on top of the lasagna. Adjust for salt and add more cayenne if you want.

Heat a large pot of water and cook lasagna according to directions on the package. Drain and cool a bit.

Coat the bottom of a 9-inch by 11-inch baking dish with a bit of the sauce and add a layer of the lasagna. Cover with some sauce, some of the ricotta, and some of the Parmesan. Add another layer of lasagna and repeat. Add the third layer of lasagna and cover with the sauce and Parmesan. Cover the dish with foil to keep it from drying out and bake for 25 minutes.

Pasta Primavera

Primavera means spring. You can use almost any combination of vegetables. It is important to cook them al dente. This dish has enough flavor to work well with the whole-wheat pasta.

YIELD: SERVES 4

2 tablespoons extra-virgin olive oil

½ cup cauliflower florets, small

½ cup broccoli florets, small

1 red bell pepper, seeded, deveined, and diced

1 zucchini, sliced

½ medium onion, chopped

4 cloves garlic, finely chopped

1 small carrot, cut into 1-inch lengths and sliced vertically into thin strips

2 ribs celery, sliced thin

¼ cup fresh salsa, (Chachies "medium hot" brand recommended)

3 fresh Roma tomatoes, diced

salt, pepper, and sugar to taste

1 pound dried pasta such as spaghetti, linguini, fettuccini, or angel hair, preferably whole wheat (Whole Foods 365 brand recommended)

Parmesan cheese, grated

Heat 1 tablespoon of the olive oil in a large skillet and sauté the cauliflower, broccoli, bell pepper, zucchini, onion, garlic, carrot, and celery. Add salt and pepper, and toss frequently. When the vegetables are nearly done to the texture you want (al dente is recommended), add the tomatoes and salsa. Cook for about 5 more minutes, tossing frequently. Test for salt and add sugar if necessary.

Meanwhile cook and drain the pasta. Put into a pasta bowl, add the remaining tablespoon of olive oil, and toss. Add the vegetables and toss well again. Serve with grated Parmesan cheese.

Pasta with Bitter Leaves

This is one of my favorite pasta dishes, and is very simple to prepare. Any of the combinations of meat and leaves will work. Cook what is available and/or what you like best.

YIELD: SERVES 4

2 tablespoons extra-virgin olive oil

½–1 teaspoon red pepper flakes

1 ounce pancetta, prosciutto, or Italian sausage, finely chopped

6 cloves garlic, finely chopped

1½ cups chicken stock (preferably homemade)

salt, to taste

2 cups finely chopped dandelion greens, arugula, or radicchio

¾ pound dried pasta, or 1 pound of fresh pasta
(preferably fettuccine)

Parmesan cheese, grated

Heat 1 tablespoon of the olive oil in a large pan over medium heat. Add meat and pepper flakes. Cook over medium-low heat until meat begins to brown. Add garlic and cook about 3 more minutes. Add chicken stock and bring to fast simmer. Let the stock reduce slightly for 5 to 10 minutes. Test for salt.

Cook pasta. While pasta is cooking, add greens to stock and stir well to coat. When pasta is done, drain, and put into a pasta bowl. Toss with remaining tablespoon of olive oil. Add sauce and toss to mix the leaves and coat the pasta well. Serve with grated Parmesan.

Pasta with Garbanzo Bean Sauce

This is a very interesting and unusual dish.
Sounds strange, tastes great.

YIELD: SERVES 4

2–3 tablespoons extra-virgin olive oil

4 cloves garlic, finely chopped

½ jalapeno chili, finely chopped, or ½ teaspoon
crushed red pepper flakes

4 tablespoons mild or medium salsa (preferably fresh)

1 16-ounce can garbanzo beans, rinsed and drained

4 cups hot water

salt and pepper, to taste

½ pound dry fettuccine or other pasta,
broken into short lengths

Parmesan cheese, grated

Heat the olive oil in a large non-stick skillet over medium heat. Add the garlic and jalapeno. Cook over medium heat until the garlic turns golden.

Meanwhile, place the salsa, half the garbanzo beans, and about 2 cups hot water in a blender, and purée. Add the purée to the skillet and bring to a slow boil. Add the pasta and remaining garbanzos to the pan. Test for salt. Simmer, stirring frequently. Add hot water as necessary to maintain the consistency, until the pasta is cooked to your taste. As the pasta cooks, the sauce will thicken and blend. Cooking the pasta takes about 15 to 25 minutes. Serve with grated Parmesan cheese on the side.

Pasta with Seafood

This dish is wonderful with fresh pasta.
My wife told me not to make it, because she would not like it.
After the meal she said it was the best pasta she ever had.

YIELD: SERVES 4–6

2 tablespoons extra-virgin olive oil

5 scallions, finely chopped

4–6 cloves garlic, finely chopped

½ jalapeno chili, finely chopped

2 ribs celery, chopped

½ cup dry white wine

5–6 fresh Roma tomatoes, diced in 1-inch pieces
(substitute any ripe tomatoes)

8–10 basil leaves, shredded

salt and pepper to taste

About 1 teaspoon sugar, depending on sweetness
of the tomatoes

½ pound fish fillets such as Tilapia in ¾-inch dice
(any firm white fish will do)

1 pound fettuccine or other wide pasta, preferably fresh

Parmesan cheese, grated

Sauté the scallions, garlic, jalapeno, and celery in 1 tablespoon of the olive oil until they soften. Add wine and cook for about 5 more minutes. Add tomatoes, basil, salt, and pepper and cook until a sauce begins to form, 10 to 15 minutes. Adjust for salt, and add sugar if necessary. Add fish and cook slowly until just done. Meanwhile, cook the pasta. Toss the pasta with remaining tablespoon of olive oil and sauce, and serve with Parmesan cheese on the side.

Pasta with Sausage and Tomatoes

This is simple to prepare, and very good. My local market makes a nice chicken jalapeno sausage that is perfect. A hot turkey Italian sausage would work well also.

YIELD: SERVES 4–6

2 tablespoons extra-virgin olive oil

½–1 pound chicken or turkey sausage,
cut into ¾-inch pieces

½–1 teaspoon crushed red pepper flakes
(omit if using hot sausage)

2–3 ribs celery, chopped

1 medium onion, chopped

4–6 cloves garlic, finely chopped

6–8 fresh Roma tomatoes, diced into 1-inch pieces
(substitute any ripe tomatoes)

1 teaspoon sugar

salt and pepper, to taste

1 pound fettuccini (preferably fresh, but, dried wide
pastas will also work)

Parmesan cheese, grated

Heat 1 tablespoon olive oil in a saucepan over medium heat. Add sausage and pepper flakes. When sausage begins to brown, add celery and onions. When onion is translucent, add garlic and cook about two more minutes. Then add tomatoes, sugar, salt, and pepper. Cook over low heat until tomatoes begin to break apart, about 30 to 60 minutes. Cook pasta, drain, put into a pasta bowl and toss with the remaining tablespoon of sauce. Serve with grated Parmesan cheese.

Thai-style Pasta

*Asian pasta is great too. There are many kinds of noodles,
including wheat noodles, buckwheat noodles (soba), and rice
noodles. Here is another simple dish with a spicy taste.*

YIELD: SERVES 4

3 tablespoons smooth peanut butter
(made without hydrogenated oils or sugar)

1–2 tablespoons soy sauce

1–2 tablespoons fresh lemon juice

1 tablespoon sugar

$\frac{1}{2}$ cup hot water

2 tablespoons canola oil

4 cloves garlic, finely chopped

$\frac{1}{2}$–1 jalapeno chili, finely chopped

1 tablespoon fresh ginger, finely chopped

1 pound dried Asian or Italian noodles

$\frac{1}{2}$ cup roasted Spanish peanuts, for garnish

Mix the peanut butter, soy sauce (to taste), lemon juice, sugar, and hot
water in a small bowl, until peanut butter is incorporated.

Heat the canola oil in a large skillet over medium-high heat. Add the garlic,
jalapeno, and ginger. Cook for 2 minutes. Add the sauce, lower the heat,
and mix well. Add water to the sauce if it gets too thick. Adjust for salt,
sugar, and lemon.

Cook the noodles, and drain. Toss with the sauce, garnish with peanuts, and
serve.

Pasta Bolognese

This recipe is adapted from the classic recipe from Marcella Hazan's Essentials of Classic Italian Cooking. *However, she recommends a fatty cut of ground beef, such as chuck, and would not likely be comfortable with my version, which is much lower in fat, but still very good.*

YIELD: SERVES 4

3 tablespoons olive oil, divided

½ cup onion, chopped

⅔ cup celery, chopped

⅔ cup carrot, chopped

¾ pound ground turkey

salt and freshly ground black pepper, to taste

1 cup whole milk

⅛ teaspoon nutmeg, freshly ground

1 cup dry white wine such as Chardonnay, Sauvignon Blanc,
or Pinot Grigio

1 can (28 ounces) plum tomatoes (imported Italian are best),
cut up with their juices

2 pounds fresh pasta or 1 pound dried pasta
(a wide pasta such as tagliatelle is best)

Parmesan cheese, freshly grated

This is best cooked in a very heavy pot. I have an enameled cast-iron pot that I use especially for this dish. Add 2 tablespoons of the oil and onion and turn the heat on medium. When the onions are translucent, add the celery and carrot and cook for about 2 minutes, stirring to coat the vegetables. Add the turkey, about $1/2$ teaspoon of salt, and a dash of fresh ground pepper. Cook until the meat has lost its red color, crumbling it. Add the milk, lower the heat and simmer until it is completely evaporated, about 20 minutes. Stir occasionally. Add nutmeg. Add the wine and simmer about 20 minutes until it has evaporated. Add the tomatoes and mix well.

When the sauce begins to bubble, reduce the heat so that the sauce barely simmers, with only occasional bubbles. Cook uncovered for at least three hours, stirring periodically. If the sauce begins to dry out, small amounts of water may be added. At the end, the fat must separate from the sauce. (It is the fat that will ensure the coating of all the pasta.) Adjust for salt.

At around three hours, the consistency of the sauce changes dramatically. You have a ragu rather than cooked meat and tomatoes.

Cook the pasta, drain, and place it in a pasta bowl. Toss with 1 tablespoon of olive oil. Add the sauce, and toss until all of the pasta is coated.

VEGETABLES AND SIDE DISHES

Braised Greens

This is a very healthy dish. Do not overcook.
The leaves should retain some texture.

YIELD: SERVES 4

1–2 tablespoons extra-virgin olive oil

½ ounce pancetta or bacon, in ¼-inch dice (optional)

4–6 cloves garlic, finely chopped

1 bunch (about 1 pound) of Swiss chard, kale, collard greens,
or dandelion greens, shredded into 1-inch wide strips

½ cup Panko-style breadcrumbs (optional)

salt and pepper, to taste

½ lemon, juiced (optional)

In a large, deep skillet with a lid, heat the oil and sauté the bacon until nearly done. Add the garlic and cook for 2 to 3 minutes. Add the greens and sauté briefly, tossing to coat them with oil over medium heat. Toss with the breadcrumbs. Cover and lower the heat. Cook for 5 to 10 minutes, until tender. Add salt, pepper, and lemon juice to taste, then serve.

Variation: These greens are also good braised without the pancetta and breadcrumbs. After shredding the greens, place them in a steamer and steam for 15 to 20 minutes. Add the garlic and cook for 2 to 3 minutes. Add salt, pepper, and lemon juice, then serve.

Baked Potatoes

The quality of a baked potato depends, more than anything, on the quality of the potatoes you buy. Our local organic market, Jimbo's, has potatoes that taste much better than those I get from any other local store. The produce manager at Jimbo's believes that they are better because they are certified organic, which requires more care and attention from the farmer. He does not believe they are fresher than the potatoes in the supermarkets. He recommends Grade A, which are the larger potatoes with no scarring.

Russet potatoes, scrubbed and dried

olive oil

salt and pepper, to taste

Preheat the oven to 375°F. Puncture the skin of each potato with the tip of a knife, all around, about 1 to 2 inches apart, to enable steam to escape in baking. Coat the potatoes with a little olive oil, and place them in a baking dish. Bake until done, at least one hour. Test for doneness by inserting a knife. The knife should slide in to the center easily.

Serve with olive oil (instead of butter) on the side, salt, and pepper. When the potatoes are cooked in this way, the skin is the best part.

Hash-Browned Potatoes

This is a wonderful dish when made with good potatoes.

YIELD: SERVES 4

6 medium Yukon Gold, or other waxy potatoes

2 to 3 tablespoons extra-virgin olive oil

1 medium red onion, chopped

salt and pepper, to taste

Boil the potatoes until nearly done. Remove from water and cool, and then slice. If you overcook the potatoes, they will crumble during frying. The dish will still be edible, but not as nice.

Heat oil in a heavy skillet over medium heat. Add onions and cook for about 2 minutes. Then add the potatoes. Salt and pepper to taste. Cook, tossing frequently, until potatoes are browned making sure they are fully cooked.

Mashed Potatoes

This recipe is a starting point. You can add a variety of seasonings, like minced garlic or minced fresh fennel, depending upon your taste.

YIELD: SERVES 4–6

2 pounds Yukon Gold or Yellow Finn potatoes, scrubbed and cut into 2-inch pieces

4 tablespoons extra-virgin olive oil

$1\frac{1}{2}$ cups low-fat milk

1 cup cooked frozen or fresh corn

salt and pepper, to taste

Boil potatoes until done. Drain and place in bowl. Begin to mash with potato masher or in a mixer at low speed. Add oil and mash a bit more. Add milk, salt, and pepper. Mash until all liquid is absorbed and the mixture is relatively smooth. Mix in corn. Test for salt and pepper, then serve.

Sautéed Brussels Sprouts

I used to think I did not like Brussels sprouts. It turned out that I just did not know how to cook them. This is a simple and wonderful dish if you can get good sprouts. The oil, garlic, and pancetta complement the flavor of the sprouts. If they are very large (about the size of golf balls) cut them in half.

YIELD: SERVES 4–6

2 pounds Brussels sprouts, washed and trimmed

1½ tablespoons extra-virgin olive oil

3 cloves garlic, finely chopped

1 ounce pancetta, finely chopped (optional)

Place the sprouts in a bowl, uncovered, and microwave for 2 minutes. Alternatively, place in boiling water for 4 minutes. Without this step, it is very difficult to get them cooked through in a sauté pan. Drain and place in a sauté pan with the olive oil, garlic, and pancetta if using. Sauté over medium heat until the sprouts are browned in spots and cooked through. This takes about 20 minutes. Serve immediately, pouring the oil and cooked garlic from the pan over the sprouts.

Braised Rapini (Broccoli Rabe)

This is similar to the previous recipe, but uses broth to sweeten
the bitter rapini. The rapini has plenty of flavor,
so you do not need garlic or pancetta.

YIELD: SERVES 4

2 bunches rapini (about 1 pound)

1–2 tablespoons extra-virgin olive oil

½ cup chicken stock (preferably homemade)

salt and pepper, to taste

Shred the rapini into 1-inch wide strips. In a large, deep skillet with a lid, heat the oil. Add the greens and sauté briefly, tossing to coat them with oil over medium heat. Add the chicken stock, cover, lower the heat, and cook for 10 to 15 minutes. Add salt and pepper to taste, then serve.

SALAD STUFF

Zesty Vinegar and Oil Salad Dressing

This is a very simple way to make a delicious dressing for fresh salads. My local organic market sells an herb dressing that I sometimes use in place of the fresh salsa, or even along with it. When making enough for just one salad, I never worry about creating an elegant emulsion of the olive oil and vinegar. After all, you can dress a salad effectively by pouring on the oil, tossing, and then adding the vinegar.

YIELD: MAKES ENOUGH DRESSING FOR A SALAD TO FEED FOUR

3 tablespoons extra-virgin olive oil

1 to 1½ tablespoons white wine vinegar to taste

1 teaspoon salt

1 teaspoon sugar

2 tablespoons fresh salsa (found in the deli section of most supermarkets)

Combine ingredients in a small bowl or cup and mix well. Test for salt, sugar, and vinegar. Pour onto salad and toss well.

Chef's Salad

This is really a concept rather than a recipe. The basics are lettuce and dressing. I suggest using a lettuce or a mixture of lettuces other than iceberg, which is the least nutritious of all lettuces. Choose ingredients from the list, based on what you like and what is available. Quantities are almost entirely optional, but you want enough lettuce so that the mixture is not too dense. This makes an excellent meal, especially on a warm day.

Lettuce

Bibb, Boston, or romaine with shredded bitter leaves
such as radicchio, arugula, watercress, spinach,
curly endive, escarole, or mustard greens

Meat/Dairy

chicken, turkey, and/or cheese, sliced into julienne strips

Vegetable/Fruits

avocado, peeled and chopped

garbanzo beans, red kidney beans, white beans (soaked, cooked, and rinsed,
or from can)

beets, sliced or diced

carrot, peeled and chopped

celery, chopped

fennel bulb, chopped

green beans, chopped

cucumber, peeled, seeded, and diced

red, yellow, or green pepper, seeded and diced

onion, sliced or chopped

tomatoes, diced

Fresh Herbs

basil, Italian parsley, finely chopped

Nuts and Seeds

walnuts, pine nuts, or others

Dried Fruit

raisins, cranberries, or others

Other

salad dressing (use recipe from page 179)

croutons (watch out for trans fat in store-bought)

Mix the ingredients to your particular taste, toss with dressing, and serve with crusty whole-grain bread.

Tabbouli

Necessity is the mother of invention. I was making this and discovered I was out of lemons. I tried a grapefruit. I still needed to go out for a lemon, but the grapefruit juice gave it a wonderful flavor.

YIELD: SERVES 4

1 cup bulgur wheat

1–1½ cups boiling water

1 grapefruit, juiced

1 or 2 lemons, juiced

¼ cup extra-virgin olive oil

½ teaspoon salt

½ red onion, finely chopped

1 cup Italian parsley, chopped

1 cucumber, peeled, seeded, and diced

2 Roma tomatoes, diced

Place the bulgur in a large bowl, pour in the boiling water, then allow to stand at room temperature for about 1 hour, until the bulgur has softened. If you have a fine sieve, use it to extract any remaining water from the bulgur. Place the bulgur in a bowl and mix in the remaining ingredients. Adjust for salt and lemon juice. Refrigerate for at least 1 hour before serving.

Tomato and Basil Salad

This is a light, tasty first course.
Remember, tomatoes are a fruit.

YIELD: SERVES 4

4 medium tomatoes, sliced

12 fresh basil leaves, approximate

½ red onion, finely chopped

olive oil

Balsamic vinegar

salt and pepper, to taste

Arrange tomato slices on four plates. Top with basil leaves and onion, then drizzle with olive oil and vinegar. Sprinkle with salt and pepper. Serve immediately.

Tuna Salad

*Mayonnaise is not a requirement for an excellent tuna salad.
If you must include it, use a canola oil or olive oil
mayonnaise with no trans fat.*

Yield: Makes enough for 3–4 sandwiches

1 can (6-ounces) tuna, packed in water or olive oil

¼ cup red onion, finely chopped

1½ tablespoons sweet pickle relish

1 tablespoon red or white wine vinegar

1 tablespoon extra-virgin olive oil
(or less if tuna is packed in oil)

salt and pepper, to taste

tomato, sliced for garnish

lettuce, torn into leaves for garnish

Drain tuna, if using water pack. Mix all ingredients with a fork, breaking tuna apart until the ingredients are mixed well. Serve either on toasted whole-wheat bread with lettuce and tomato or over sliced tomatoes on a bed of lettuce.

Calamari in Beet Sauce

*This recipe is adapted from one sent to me by Alain Genchi,
the chef at Barra Azul (The Blue Bar), one of my favorite
restaurants in Ensenada. The trick is to get the beets and
calamari both done properly. The beets should be a bit
al dente and the calamari should not be overcooked.
It is also a wonderful appetizer served warm or cold.*

YIELD: SERVES 4

2 tablespoons extra-virgin olive oil

3 cloves garlic, finely chopped

1 teaspoon fresh ginger, finely chopped

½ serrano chili, finely chopped

1 cup beets, chopped

½ pound calamari (squid), cleaned and chopped

½ cup dry white wine

½ cup orange juice

salt, pepper, and sugar, to taste

Heat olive oil in pan and sauté the garlic, ginger, serrano, and beets until
the garlic begins to soften, about 5 minutes. Add the calamari and sauté
about 3 more minutes. Then add the wine and orange juice. Bring to a boil,
then reduce heat and simmer until the beets are cooked al dente, about 4
minutes. Add salt, pepper, and sugar to taste. Serve immediately or chill it
in the refrigerator for 1 hour and then serve.

Asian Slaw

This is a simple salad with lots of flavor.

YIELD: SERVES 4

1 medium head green or red cabbage, shredded

1 carrot, grated

½ cup seasoned rice vinegar

½ cup fresh cilantro, chopped

1 tablespoon sesame oil

½ cup peanuts

salt and pepper, to taste

Place all ingredients in a bowl and toss thoroughly to coat. Adjust for salt and pepper. Cover and chill at least 1 hour. Toss again before serving.

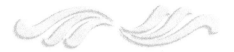

Epilogue

I HAVE BEEN AT WORK ON THIS BOOK for nearly three years. It has been a period of education for me, as well as increased awareness. Every day I scan the online versions of the *New York Times,* the *Washington Post,* the *Los Angeles Times, and* the Sunday *New York Times.* Almost daily, one of these papers has an article on diet and health. Although there is still the occasional "SEVEN DAYS TO A THINNER YOU" type of article, there is more and more serious content. While I have not done a statistical study, I perceive a trend.

For example, the *Washington Post's* June 19, 2007 edition featured an article headlined "JAPAN'S NEW PUBLIC HEALTH PROBLEM IS GETTING BIG: OBESITY HAS GROWN—ALONG WITH APPETITE FOR WESTERN FOOD." The article describes how Japan, once a paragon of leanness, is developing an obesity problem, with an alarming rate of obesity in children that reached 24.3 percent in 2005. The article blames the problem on the increasing popularity of Western food with its high content of saturated fat. It further claims that the Japanese are not eating more calories, but are simply eating the wrong kinds of food. Surveys of Greece and Southern Italy show a similar trend. Overweight, obesity, and heart disease are on the rise worldwide. The culprits cited are almost always Western food and a more sedentary lifestyle.

Along with this trend of increasing obesity is a trend of increasing concern. That is what gives rise to the frequent articles in the popular media. There is at least a segment of our population that is very concerned about this public health problem. Virtually every major newspaper runs regular articles on weight loss. CNN's chief medical correspondent, Dr. Sanjay Gupta, has completed his second annual nationwide tour to fight the epidemic of obesity.

At the local level, New York City has taken the extraordinary step of banning trans fat, requiring restaurants to phase it out by July 2008. Certainly there remains the threat that the regulation will not be enforced, or that industry will obtain federal or state legislation to invalidate the local ordinance." In the meantime, it is a significant statement.

Another example of this concern at the local level involves my younger son and his partner. My son's business sells food to school lunch programs. As his awareness has grown, he has become increasingly concerned about what they are selling. The most popular products in this market are chicken nuggets, pizza, and burritos. Typically these are loaded with saturated fat and refined carbohydrates. Most of the products are very high in sodium, and many contain trans fat. My son and his partner are developing and selling healthy alternatives. They are focusing on tasty foods made from healthier ingredients without trans fats. For example, they offer burritos and pizza made with whole wheat and chicken that is not treated with sodium. Although the program is very new, it has generated strong interest in the local community.

We have increasing concern on national and local levels about the huge public health problem of obesity, heart disease, and type 2 diabetes. This is reflected in the media, in actions at the local level, and in the marketplace.

A CLASH OF TWO CULTURES

Along with this trend of increasing awareness, there are powerful industries that are trying to enrich their shareholders by increasing their sales. Much of those sales are generated from products very high in saturated fat and refined carbohydrates. If you are used to eating a lot of saturated fat, the taste is very appealing. Refined carbohydrates are very convenient, especially for the marketer. They taste good and have a long shelf life. One of the most widely used refined carbohydrates is high-fructose corn syrup (HFCS). I have discussed in Chapter 2 the controversy specific to HFCS. It may be worse than the sucrose (table sugar) it replaced. Even if it is no worse, we have seen a dramatic and unfortunate increase in the amount of sugar we consume.

The fast-food industry is still dominated by burgers and sodas, along with fries cooked in trans fat. This industry is very aggressive at marketing, especially to young children. An exception in terms of nutrition is the restaurant chain Subway, which positions itself as a healthy alternative. And as you can read in Chapter 7, they do offer some relatively healthy alternatives.

The dairy industry is still trying to convince us that we "never outgrow our need for milk," butter, cheese, and ice cream, too. These foods are all very high in saturated fat, and the ice cream contains lots of sugar or HFCS. The industry still has many school programs that push milk to the kids. According to the National Dairy Council, 5.2 billion half pints of milk were served in school nutrition programs in 2002. To qualify for federal reimbursement, a school lunch must include milk. This may be a good idea in areas where there is nutritional deprivation. In my grammar school, which was not nutritionally deprived, I was under considerable pressure to drink my daily lukewarm half pint of milk, which I hated and resisted.

The soft drink industry does its part. While suffering a slight decline, U.S. soft drink sales exceeded 10 billion cases in 2005. The bulk of this is in the traditional, HFCS-laced sodas. Coke Classic and Pepsi alone account for nearly 3 billion cases of soda sold.

Finally, we have the food-processing industry, providing everything from breakfast cereals to midnight snacks. Much of this food is full of saturated fat, trans fat, and sugar, typically in the form of HFCS. Their goal would appear to be getting the maximum appeal for the minimum cost, essentially independent of what it takes to get here. Certainly, we see more products advertising "0 trans fat," "low fat," and "low carb." But these are taking advantage of trends, not setting them. Every one of these industries is supported by sophisticated marketing efforts, and much of the marketing is to kids. Moreover, a thorough examination of the nutrition panels of these offerings usually describes a product that is far from ideal from a health standpoint.

So we have two forces in conflict: 1) a growing public concern about the serious problem of obesity and related conditions that include cardiovascular disease and type 2 diabetes; and 2) a collection of industrial giants that happen to be promoting foods that contribute to this problem. On the side of the industries are creative marketers. They stress image, convenience, value, and flavor. They capture shelf space and promote with discounts, coupons, and more food for the same price. Value (meaning how many tasty calories you get for your money) is very important. Attempting to deal with the public health problem are an increasing number of health authorities, and a growing culture of what are essentially advocates of healthier eating, and healthier lifestyles. This latter group is very diverse, ranging from devout vegetarians to buyers of organic foods. It also includes the growing legion of fitness enthusiasts—joggers, cyclists, spin-class mavens, yoga students, ad infinitum.

I view this as a clash of two cultures. This conflict can be clearly illustrated by a useful oversimplification. On the one side, we have the mall culture of convenience and fast food. The mall is reached by car. The only exercise is walking from store to store. The food court dependably offers high-fat, highly refined carbohydrate fare. There is enormous uniformity and predictability in the stores. The whole thing works particularly well if you are in a hurry. You always know what is there and where to find it. Once you are inside, it is hard to tell whether you are in Seattle or Orlando.

On the other side, we have a health and fitness culture. It involves a different set of activities including shopping at organic markets, eschewing fast food, jogging, cycling, or working out on a regular basis. Of course, this culture is very diverse. Shopping at Whole Foods Market or any natural foods store is not much like growing your own organic produce, but both are ways to obtain healthy food. And, both are more similar to each other than either one is to a visit to a fast-food outlet or a mall food court.

THE EPICENTER OF THESE TWO CULTURES

The clash of these two cultures is nowhere more prominent than in Southern California, home of Hollywood, Disneyland, and Laguna Beach. Southern California has a Mediterranean climate, but not a Mediterranean culture. By the way, I have spent about three weeks on various Italian and Spanish regions of the Mediterranean coast, and I have yet to see a mall, although I expect there must be some. Skateboarders there must have a venue problem. Southern California is an engine of the mall culture. Virtually all of its communities are designed around the automobile. You can't walk to anything and there is virtually no public transportation. Thus, the region is dominated by malls.

Southern California is also a culture in which appearance and image are paramount, making it an engine of the health and fitness culture as well. (Of course, this also makes it an engine of cosmetic surgery.) It's climate, especially the mild climate of coastal areas like Laguna Beach, is a great facilitator of health and fitness and allows local growers to provide fresh fruits and vegetables year round.

The health and fitness culture is strong in other places, like the Bay Area in Northern California and Boulder, Colorado to name two. But in these places the mall culture is less prominent. Southern California is a battleground in which two strong forces are arrayed. They are not always consciously fighting against each other, but there is a battle going on for the hearts and minds (and mouths) of the population.

A SOUTHERN CALIFORNIA SOLUTION

The Laguna Beach Diet is an attempt to provide an approach to weight loss and better health that can appeal to both sides. The following attributes contribute to this moderate solution:

- The diet is not an ascetic solution with severe deprivation. It does not require you to endure daily spin classes or to become an ultra-marathon runner. While some people at the extreme end of the health and fitness culture might actually *prefer* a little more pain, to convince themselves that they are really accomplishing something, I think they can live with this.

- It is ethnically diverse. It incorporates a variety of foods to appeal to a variety of tastes.

- It is satisfying. Low-calorie and low-fat diets always leave one unsatisfied. This diet allows plenty of food and plenty of fat, so long as it is the right kind of fat.

- It is not expensive. Fresh fruits and vegetables and whole grains are not necessarily expensive. Rice and beans with a little chicken and a green salad make an excellent and healthy meal that is very inexpensive.

- It is convenient. While it is not burgers, fries, large sugar sodas, and cookies, you can still eat fast food with unsweetened ice tea and a little chocolate, as long as you choose carefully.

To convert to the Laguna Beach Diet does require some discipline, especially at first. If you are accustomed to burgers, fries, and sodas, you will miss them for a while. But over time, your tastes will adjust, and you will get even more enjoyment while eating a much healthier and more natural diet. As you convert, you will feel healthier and better. You will lose weight and look better. And, you will be able to stop worrying about what you eat, or whether you are eating too much. Most important, the long-term health benefits will be enormous.

In our family, this is no longer a "diet," it is a way of life. We do not think much about the principles any longer, we just crave the right food. And by the way, our guests love our meals, too.

Selected References

Barsh GS, IS Faroogi, and S O'Rahilly. "Genetics of body-weight regulation." *Nature* 2000; 404, 644–651.

Basciano H, L Federico, and K Adeli. "Fructose, insulin resistance, and metabolic dyslipidemia." *Nutrition and Metabolism* 2005; 186: 1743–1775.

Blundell JE and NA King. "Physical activity and regulation of food intake: current evidence [roundtable consensus statement]." *Medicine and Science in Sports and Exercise* 1999; 31: S573–583.

Bray GA, SJ Nielsen, and BM Popkin. "Consumption of high-fructose corn syrup in beverages may play a role in the epidemic of obesity." *American Journal of Clinical Nutrition* 2004; 79: 537–543.

Campbell, TC and TM Campbell. *The China Study.* Dallas, TX: Benbella Books, 2004.

Esposito K, R Marfella, M Ciotola, et al. "Effect of a Mediterranean-style diet on endothelial dysfunction and markers of vascular inflammation in the metabolic syndrome." *Journal of the American Medical Association* 2004; 292: 1440–1446.

Goff SL, JM Foody, S Inzucchi, et al. "Nutrition and weight loss information in a popular diet book: is it fact, fiction, or something in between?" *Journal of General Internal Medicine* 21, 769–774, 2006.

Gonzales MA and AS Sanchez-Villegas. "The emerging role of Mediterranean diets in cardiovascular epidemiology: monounsaturated fats, olive oil, red wine or the whole pattern." *European Journal of Epidemiology* 2004; 19: 9–13.

Hadler, N. *The Last Well Person.* Montreal: McGill-Queen's University Press, 2004.

Heshka S, JW Anderson, RL Atkinson, et al. "Weight loss with self-help compared with a structured commercial program." *Journal of the American Medical Association* 2003; 289: 1792–1799.

Jacobson, MF. "High-fructose corn syrup and the obesity epidemic." *American Journal of Clinical Nutrition* 2004; 80: 1081.

Kris-Etherton P, RH Eckel, BV Howard, et al. "Lyon Diet Heart Study: benefits of a Mediterranean-style, National Cholesterol Education Program/American Heart Association step I dietary pattern on cardiovascular disease." *Circulation* 2001; 103: 1823–1825.

Kromhout D. "Diet, lifestyle and coronary heart disease: experience from the Seven Countries Study." Paper presented to the European Society of Cardiology, August 31, 2003.

MacLean PS. "A peripheral perspective of weight regain." *American Journal of Physiology-Regulatory, Integrative, and Comparative Physiology* 2005; 288: R1447–R1449.

Panagiotakos DB, C Pitsavos, C Chrysohoou, et. al. "The epidemiology of type 2 diabetes mellitus in Greek adults: the ATTICA study." *Diabetic Medicine* 2005; 22: 1581–1588.

Peeters A, JJ Barendregt, F Willekens, et. al. "Obesity in adulthood and its consequences for life expectancy: a life-table analysis." *Annals of Internal Medicine* 2003; 138: 24–33.

President's Cancer Panel. Annual Report for 2006-2007, National Cancer Institute, http://deainfo.nci.nih.gov/ADVISORY/pcp/pcp.htm, 2007.

Rissanen A, P Hakala, L Lissner, et al. "Acquired preference especially for dietary fat and obesity: a study of weight discordant monozygotic twin pairs." *International Journal of Obesity* 2002; 26: 973–977.

Scarmeas N, Y Stern, R Mayeux, et. al. "Mediterranean Diet, Alzheimer's disease, and vascular mediation." *Archives of Neurology* 2006; 63: 1709–1717.

Wansink B, MM Cheney, and N Chan. "Exploring comfort food preferences across age and gender." *Physiology and Behavior* 2003; 79, 739–747.

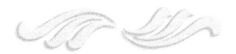

Index

About the Author

Brooks Carder was raised in Kansas and received his B.A. from Yale University and his Ph.D. in experimental psychology from the University of Pennsylvania. His career began as assistant professor of psychology at UCLA, followed by fifteen years as an executive of a drug rehabilitation organization, and ten years running a mid-sized marketing communications company. In addition, he has consulted to many of the *Fortune* 50 in the areas of quality, safety, marketing, and human resources. He has published over forty papers in scientific and professional journals, along with one book, *Measurement Matters: How Effective Measurement Drives Business and Safety Performance* (Milwaukee, WI: ASQ Press, 2004). He currently lives with his wife and chief food critic, Fran, along with three shelties, and one cat in Del Mar, California. He is an avid grandparent, cook, and golfer.

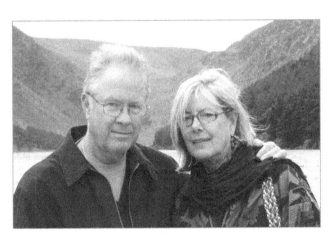

Author Brooks Carder and his wife, Fran, at Glendaloch, outside of Dublin, Ireland. *(Photo courtesy of Brooks Carder.)*

Printed in the USA
CPSIA information can be obtained
at www.ICGtesting.com
JSHW012029140824
68134JS00033B/2946